MATCHA
A COOKBOOK

First published in Great Britain in 2018
by Aster, an imprint of
Octopus Publishing Group Ltd
Carmelite House
50 Victoria Embankment
London EC4Y 0DZ
www.octopusbooks.co.uk

An Hachette UK Company
www.hachette.co.uk

The authorized representative in the EEA
is Hachette Ireland, 8 Castlecourt Centre,
Dublin 15, D15 XTP3, Ireland
(email: info@hbgi.ie)

This edition published in 2026

Copyright © Octopus Publishing
Group Ltd 2018, 2026

Distributed in the US by Hachette
Book Group
1290 Avenue of the Americas
4th and 5th Floors, New York, NY 10104

Distributed in Canada by Canadian
Manda Group, 664 Annette St.,
Toronto, Ontario, Canada M6S 2C8

All rights reserved. No part of this work
may be reproduced or utilized in any
form or by any means, electronic or
mechanical, including photocopying,
recording or by any information storage
and retrieval system, without the prior
written permission of the publisher.

ISBN: 978-0-6006-4010-3
eISBN: 978-0-6006-4011-0

A CIP catalogue record for this book
is available from the British Library.

Printed and bound in China.

10 9 8 7 6 5 4 3 2 1

Publisher: Lucy Pessell
Senior Editor: Tim Leng
Designers: Isobel Platt & Kath Anderson
Assistant Editor: Samina Rahman
Production Controller: Allison Gonsalves

Photographer: Issy Croker
Props Stylist: Emily Ezekiel
Page 7 picture credit: Franz Eugen Köhler,
Köhler's Medizinal-Pflanzen, 1897/
Wikipedia

This FSC® label means that materials
used for the product have been
responsibly sourced.

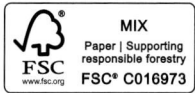

MATCHA
A COOKBOOK

Breakfast – lunch – dinner
and everything in between

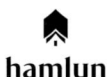

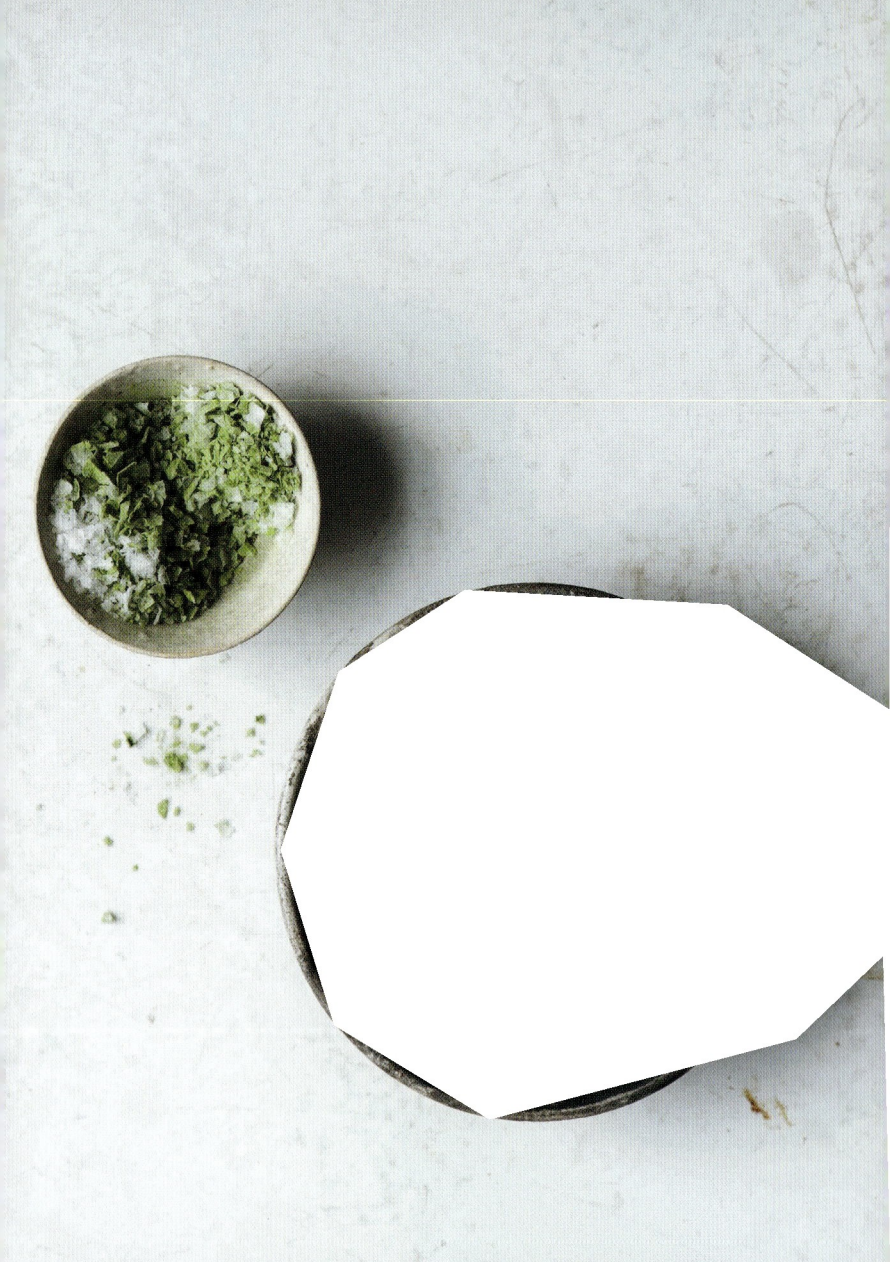

CONTENTS

7   Introduction

12 **Breakfasts**

24 **Soups, sides & snacks**

44 **Main dishes**

60 **Sweets & drinks**

78 Index

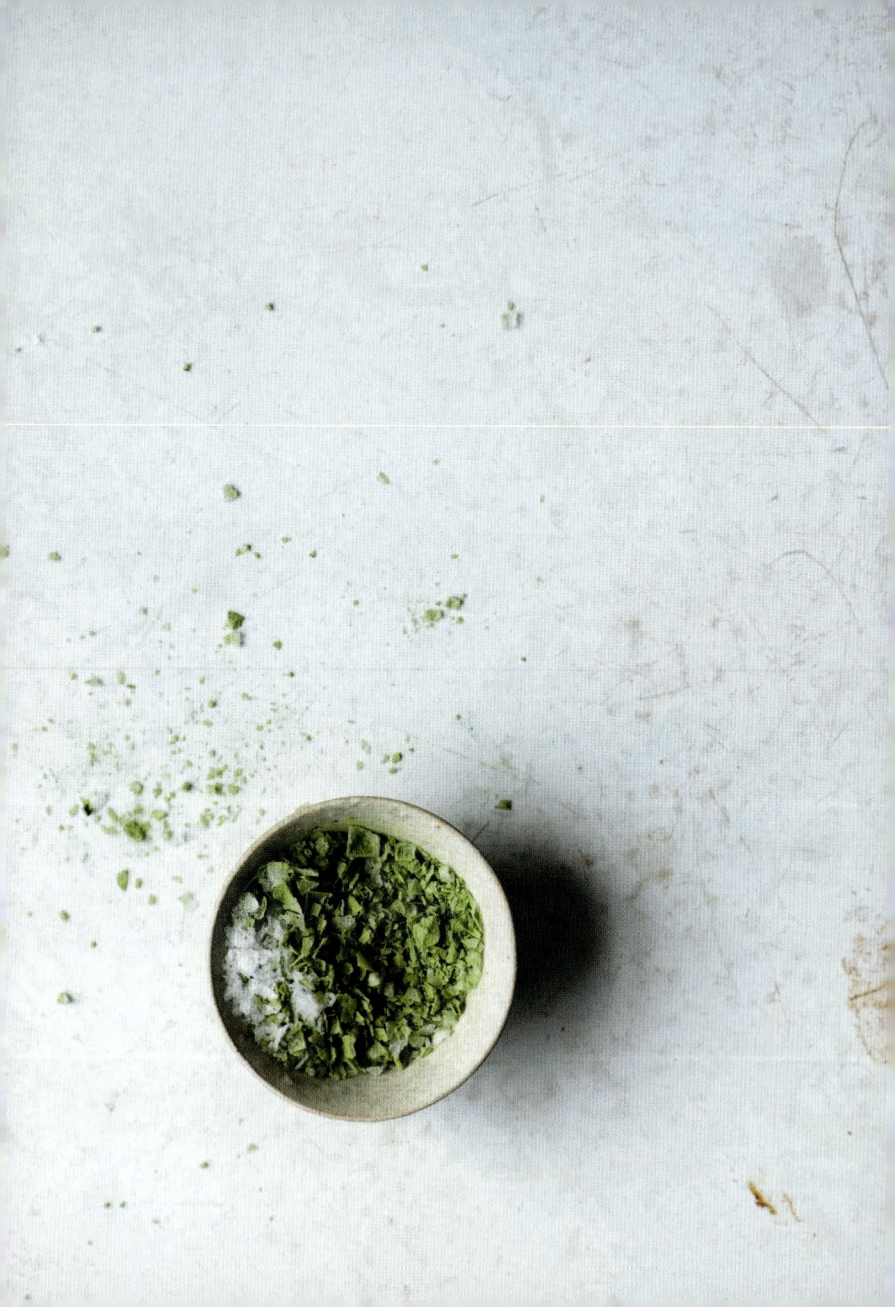

INTRODUCTION

Matcha is a fine powder made from young green tea leaves. It comes from the tea plant *Camellia sinensis*, a shrub native to southern China. In Japanese, *cha* means 'tea' and *ma* means 'powder', so the word translates literally as powdered tea. Matcha tea is therefore different from most teas, including green, that 'steep' the leaves in hot water. With matcha tea, the whole leaf is consumed.

It is believed that the first green tea seeds were brought to Japan from China by the Zen monk Eisai in 1191 AD. With the tea grown from these seeds, which he planted in Kyoto, Eisai introduced a new way of drinking tea, which became known as the matcha style. He also wrote the book *Kissa Yojoki* on the health benefits of tea, claiming that it promoted longevity, which popularized matcha tea in Japan at that time. Tea leaves had been consumed as a medicine before this, but it was Eisai who popularized the drinking of matcha tea.

The early beginnings of matcha in Japan explain why it is often associated with Zen philosophy, and in particular the Japanese tea ceremony, which celebrates beauty in simplicity and ordinary things and encourages participants to bring themselves absolutely into the present moment by focusing on the drinking of tea.

Even before the tea ceremony became a popular Zen practice, monks would drink matcha before meditating as it gave them a feeling of relaxed alertness. And historically, Samurai warriors drank the tea for its energizing properties. Now, in modern-day Japan, students will often drink matcha tea before exams for that same relaxed alertness, maintaining their energy while studying and focus during the exams.

Right: Camellia sinensis

'Tea is the ultimate mental and medical remedy and has the ability to make one's life more full and complete.'

– Myoan Eisai, *Kissa Yojoki: How to Stay Healthy by Drinking Tea*

THE HEALTH BENEFITS OF MATCHA

The positive effects felt by Zen monks and Samurai warriors many centuries ago, and so intuitively felt to be health benefits associated with drinking matcha tea, are now being supported by modern science.

All green tea is high in antioxidants due to its lack of processing; the reason matcha is considered such a powerhouse of health is because the entire leaf is consumed in the powder form, making it the most potent of all the green teas.

Matcha contains small amounts of various vitamins and minerals, but is most prized for being rich in polyphenol compounds called catechins, a type of antioxidant. As matcha is made from ground-up whole tea leaves, it is a more potent source of catechins than standard green tea, which is consumed as an infusion from which the leaves are discarded. One study found that matcha contains three times more of the catechins called epigallocatechin gallate (EGCG) – an antioxidant linked to fighting cancer, viruses and heart disease – than other standard kinds of green tea. Antioxidants are the body's defence agents and they help prevent ageing and chronic diseases. The following are all health benefits associated with matcha tea.

1. May Help Prevent Cancer
Research has shown that green tea consumption can reduce the risk of certain cancers. Among those where risk reduction has been scientifically demonstrated are bladder cancer, breast cancer, colon cancer and prostate cancer.

2. Promotes Heart Health
Matcha tea has been shown to be the highest food-level source of catechins, a group of anti-inflammatory antioxidants that help prevent heart disease. Green tea has also been shown to help lower LDL cholesterol levels, reducing the risk of stroke and hypertension.

3. High Levels of L-theanine for an Alert Calmness
Matcha is said to induce a feeling of alert calm due to its mix of L-theanine and caffeine. L-theanine is an amino acid that promotes alpha waves, which lead to a state of relaxed alertness. It has been shown to benefit people diagnosed with anxiety, enhancing mood as well as aiding concentration.

4. Recovery from Exercise
Studies suggest that the catechins in matcha tea can help speed recovery in athletes whose focus is high-intensity workouts, helping to reduce muscle damage.

5. Anti-Ageing
Catechins counteract the effects of free radicals from the environment, such as pollution, the sun's UV rays and chemicals, which can all cause cell damage.

THE JAPANESE TEA CEREMONY

Matcha is the tea used in the beautiful and exquisite Japanese tea ceremony, which was established around the year 1570 by the Zen master Sen-no-Rikyu.

There are four principles associated with the tea ceremony:
- Harmony (wa)
- Respect (kei)
- Purity (sei)
- Tranquillity (jaku)

In Japanese, the tea ceremony is called a *chado* or *sado*, meaning 'The Way of Tea'. This phrase is related to the Zen philosophy of humans always being somewhere along the way, always learning, rather than ever finished.

The tea ceremony traditionally takes place in a room that is designated just for the ceremony and is precisely four-and-a-half tatami mats in size, which is about nine square metres (100 sq ft). The guests enter the room and the host prepares the tea with very precise, slow movements. It will be a very plain room, so that all the attention is on the tea. The room will contain a stove in the middle and a kettle hanging from the ceiling over the stove. There will be bowls to drink from, the traditional bamboo whisk, scoops and ladle, along with tea caddies. Every object in the room is symbolic. All bowls are individually made and any imperfections are actually prized, as the tea ceremony celebrates beauty in imperfection. If a bowl is broken, it might be repaired using the practice of *kintsugi*, which means 'to repair with gold'. This is where gold powder is mixed in with the repair lacquer, thus making the repaired object even more valuable than the original.

COOKING WITH MATCHA

Vibrant green matcha lattes are probably the most well-known way of consuming matcha in the West, but recipes are now popping up on health blogs and in cooking magazines, offering increasingly creative ways of baking, blending and cooking with matcha powder. It's important to know that there are several different types or 'grades' of matcha available. The two particularly to look out for are 'ceremonial' grade and 'premium culinary' grade.

Ceremonial grade matcha is the highest quality green tea powder available. When drinking the classic matcha tea, it is best to use the ceremonial grade matcha powder. Although expensive, you only use a small amount to make a cup or bowl. It is a vibrant green colour and has a more delicate taste than other grades of matcha. This is because it is made from the youngest leaves, with the stems removed, and is stone-ground.

Culinary matcha powder is stronger in taste, which actually makes it better to combine with other flavours; it's also less expensive. Although it doesn't have quite the same vibrant green as ceremonial matcha, it still adds amazing colour to drinks, baked goods, dressings and sauces.

In terms of creating recipes with matcha, it is often a case of trying things out to see what works, although its slightly sweet, slightly bitter flavour goes well with dairy ingredients, citrus flavours, baked goods and dark chocolate. It also seems to add an extra layer to savoury dishes, from cauliflower cheese to hummus, poached chicken and fish.

BREAKFASTS

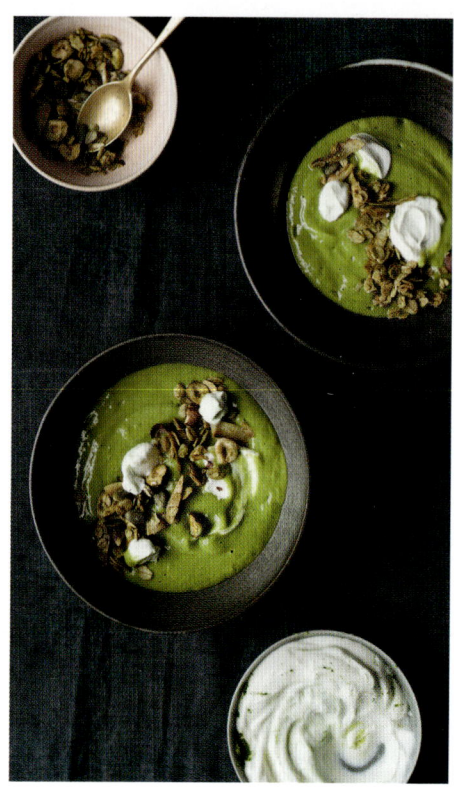

13	**Smoothie Bowl**
14	**Soda Bread**
16	**Matcha Granola**
17	**Matcha Maple Oats**
18	**Pancakes**
21	**Matcha Omelette**
22	**Eggy Bread**
23	**Matcha Scrambled Eggs**

SERVES 1

SMOOTHIE BOWL

Adding a spoonful of matcha to your morning smoothie or juice is one of the easiest ways to enjoy a daily dose of antioxidants, sharpening your focus so you're ready for the day ahead. Any 'green' smoothie or juice works well with matcha, especially with ingredients such as spinach, kale, cucumber, lime, avocado and pineapple.

½ avocado
½ banana, sliced and frozen
¼ cucumber, roughly chopped
25 g (1 oz) baby spinach leaves
50 ml (2 fl oz) coconut water
1 teaspoon matcha powder
squeeze of lime juice

TO SERVE
yogurt
Matcha Granola (see page 16)

Place all the ingredients in a blender and whizz until thick and smooth. Adjust the amount of coconut water to achieve your desired consistency.

Serve with yogurt and a sprinkling of matcha granola.

MAKES 1 SMALL LOAF

SODA BREAD

Soda bread is the easiest bread to bake as it requires no yeast. All you need to do is mix the ingredients and it's ready to go straight into the oven. The apricots in this recipe can be replaced with other dried fruit, such as raisins or cranberries, or simply omitted.

---

250 g (8 oz) spelt flour
1 teaspoon bicarbonate of soda (baking soda)
2 teaspoons matcha powder
50 g (2 oz) dried apricots, roughly chopped
200 g (7 oz) natural (plain) yogurt
splash of whole milk

Pre-heat the oven to 200°C (400°F), Gas Mark 6.

Sift the flour, bicarbonate of soda and matcha together and stir through the apricots. Form a well in the flour and add the yogurt, stirring as you pour. Bring the flour and yogurt together to form a sticky dough, adding a splash of milk if you need to.

Tip the dough on to a floured surface and knead for just a minute to form a ball before placing on a floured baking tray. Dust the dough ball, then score a deep cross in the top. Bake in the oven for 45 minutes, or until the bottom of the loaf sounds hollow when it is tapped.

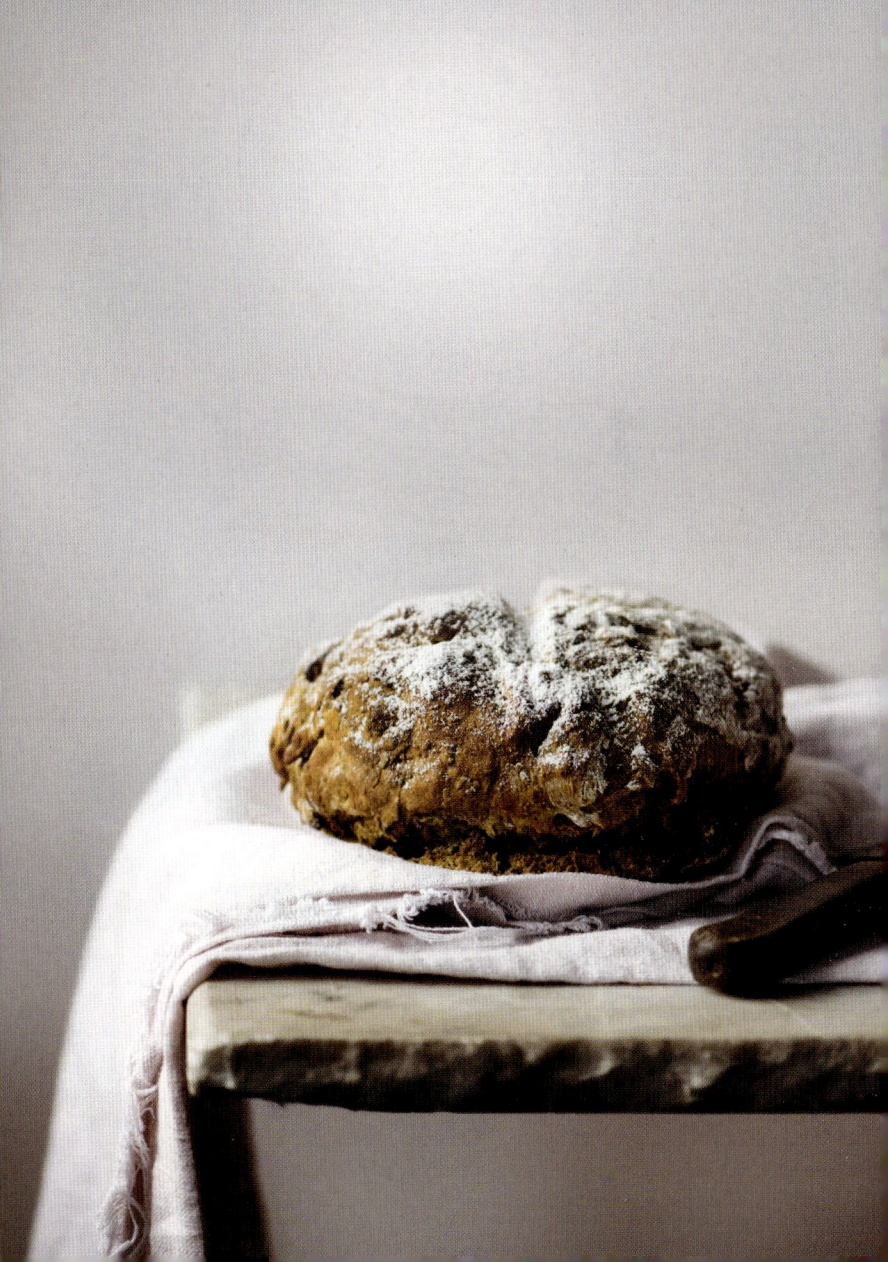

MAKES ABOUT 500 G (1 LB 2 OZ)

MATCHA GRANOLA

The Japanese discovered that matcha is a great ingredient for baking, adding a really interesting flavour, as well as the distinctive matcha colour. Since it also goes well with coconut, it makes for a really delicious nutty granola. You might also want to try making this recipe with a teaspoon of ground ginger.

---

250 g (8 oz) jumbo (old-fashioned) oats
150 g (5½ oz) hazelnuts, roughly chopped
100 g (3½ oz) dried coconut flakes
50 g (2 oz) pumpkin seeds
2 teaspoons matcha powder
2 heaped tablespoons coconut oil
3 tablespoons maple syrup
1 teaspoon vanilla extract

Preheat the oven to 140°C (275°F), Gas Mark 1 and line a large baking tray with baking paper (parchment).

Mix all the dry ingredients together in a large bowl.

Heat the coconut oil and maple syrup in a small saucepan until melted and combined, then stir in the vanilla extract. Pour this liquid into the dry ingredients and stir thoroughly so that all the oats, nuts and seeds are evenly coated.

Pour the granola into the lined baking tray and spread out evenly. Bake for about 1 hour, until golden and just crunchy. Leave to cool, then gently bring up the sides of the paper to transfer the granola to an airtight jar.

SERVES 2

MATCHA MAPLE OATS

This is such a warming way to enjoy matcha in the morning. If you soak the oats in almond milk overnight, they will be even faster to heat up for breakfast. You can use honey instead of maple syrup, and add any extra toppings you like, such as sliced bananas or berries.

---

110 g (3¾ oz) porridge (rolled) oats
½ teaspoon matcha powder
200 ml (7 fl oz) unsweetened almond milk
200 ml (7 fl oz) water
2 tablespoons maple syrup

TO SERVE
black or white sesame seeds

Put the dried oats into a saucepan and mix in the matcha. Add the almond milk along with the water and bring to the boil. Reduce the heat, cover and simmer for about 10 minutes, stirring every now and then.

Leave to stand for a couple of minutes with the lid on, then pour into bowls. Drizzle over the maple syrup and add some black or white sesame seeds to serve.

MAKES 6–8 PANCAKES

PANCAKES

Delicious on a weekend morning, these pancakes puff up really well and are a great way to enjoy quinoa flour, which, unlike most flours, is a good source of protein. You can use all quinoa flour in this recipe if you want to make gluten-free pancakes.

FOR THE PANCAKES
90 g (3 ¼ oz) quinoa flour
90 g (3 ¼ oz) spelt flour
1½ teaspoons baking powder
¼ teaspoon bicarbonate of soda (baking soda)
½ teaspoon sea salt
1 tablespoon matcha powder
1 egg
180 g (6¼ oz) Greek yogurt, plus extra to serve
250 ml (9 fl oz) whole milk (or almond milk)
1 tablespoon vanilla extract
butter or coconut oil, for frying

FOR THE BANANAS
2 bananas, halved lengthways
20 g (¾ oz) butter
2 teaspoons coconut sugar

TO SERVE
6 slices streaky (regular) bacon, fried
100 ml (3½ fl oz) maple syrup
handful of flaked almonds, toasted (optional)

Sift the quinoa and spelt flours into a large mixing bowl, add the rest of the dry ingredients and mix together thoroughly.

Beat the egg in a separate bowl and whisk in the yogurt, milk and vanilla extract. Add the wet ingredients to the dry and mix until combined into a thick batter.

Place a nonstick frying pan (skillet) over a medium heat and add a little butter or coconut oil. When melted, pour in a small ladleful of batter. Cook for about 2 minute, until you see bubbles forming on the surface, then flip over, cooking the other side for about another 2 minutes.

For the bananas, heat another pan, add the butter and, once it begins to bubble, add the sugar. When the sugar has melted, place the banana halves in the pan and turn to coat in the sugary butter. Cook on each side until caramelized.

Serve with bacon, maple syrup, Greek yogurt and flaked almonds.

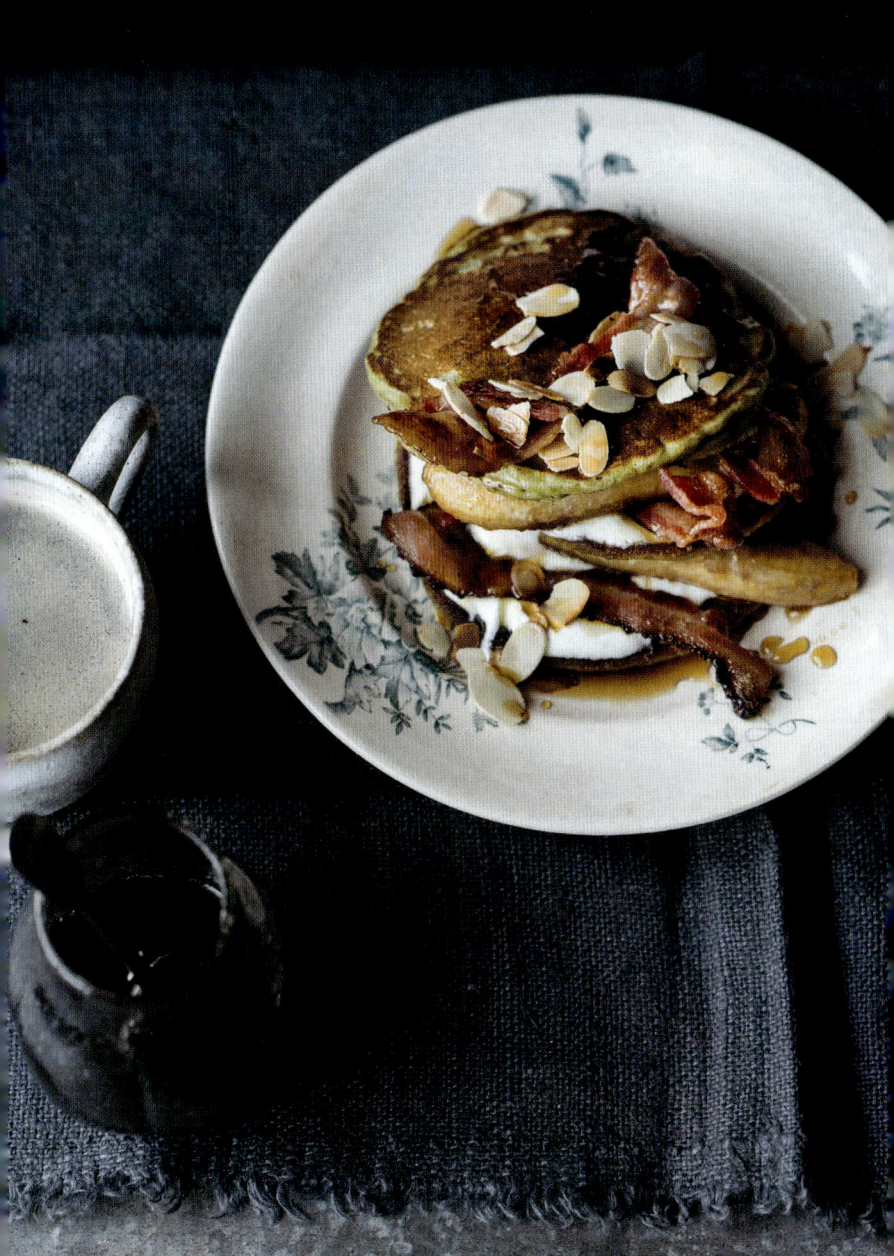

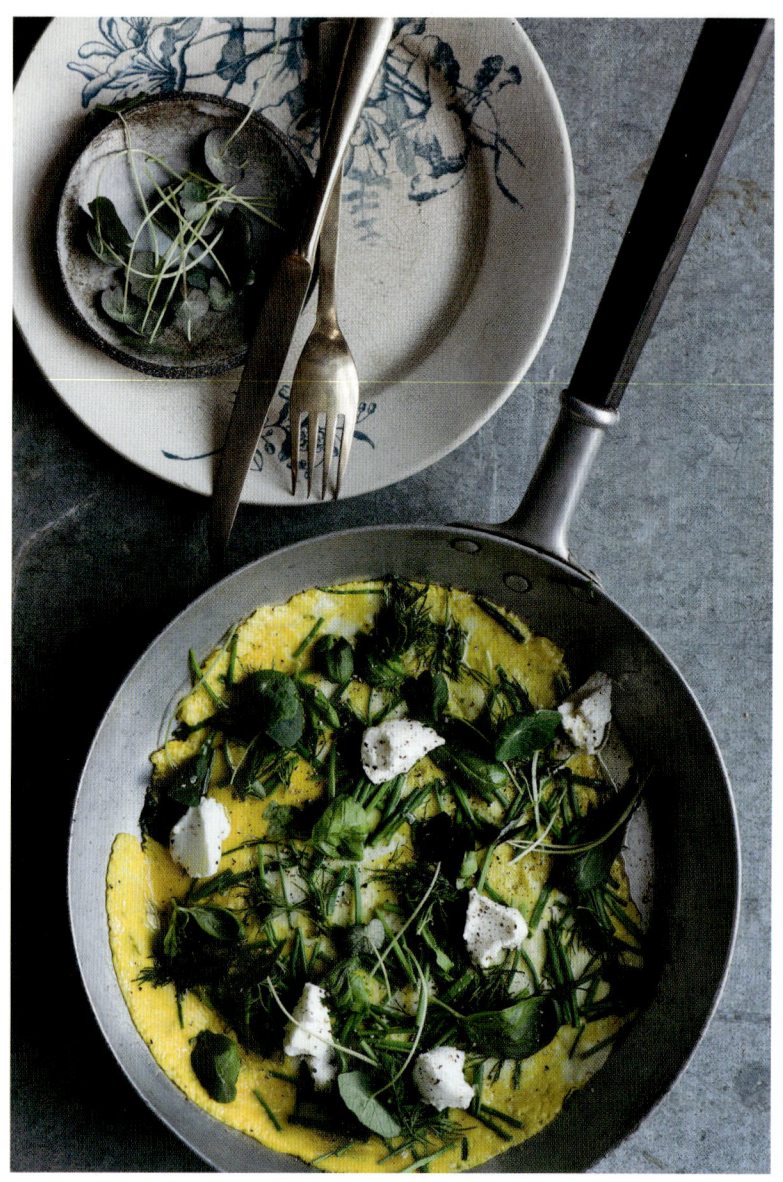

SERVES 2

MATCHA OMELETTE
with goats' cheese and herbs

The goats' cheese, soft egg omelette and generous handfuls of herbs in this recipe go brilliantly with matcha. This is a full-on breakfast packed with protein and flavour.

---

4 eggs
1 tablespoon natural (plain) yogurt
1 teaspooon matcha powder
zest of ½ lime
pinch of sea salt
10 g (¾ oz) unsalted butter
1 teaspoon olive oil
50 g (2 oz) soft goats' cheese
small handful of finely chopped mixed herbs, such as basil, dill and chives

Crack the eggs into a bowl and whisk with the yogurt, matcha powder, lime zest and salt.

Place a nonstick frying pan (skillet) over a very high heat. When it's really hot, add the butter and oil. Once the butter starts foaming, add the egg mixture.

Let the sides fluff up, pulling the edges in with a rubber spatula to allow some of the uncooked egg to run into the spaces. Dot the goats' cheese across the omelette and sprinkle with the herbs.

When the omelette is mostly cooked (the centre should still be a little runny), fold in half and slide out of the pan. Divide into two and serve immediately.

SERVES 2

EGGY BREAD
with matcha prawns

In this recipe, you make a brown matcha butter to go with the prawns and the French (or 'eggy') toast, made here with brioche. Heat the butter in the pan until it goes nutty and brown – wonderful with the lemon prawns.

---

20 g (¾ oz) unsalted butter, plus extra for frying
squeeze of lemon juice
½ teaspoon chives
½ teaspoon matcha powder
1 teaspoon coconut oil
zest of 1 lemon
12 raw tiger (jumbo) prawns
2 eggs
dash of milk
2 slices of brioche

TO SERVE
kombu, soaked
pea shoots, to garnish (optional)

The day before you want to make this, soak the kombu in cold water overnight, or for at least eight hours.

Melt the butter in a small saucepan, swirling it around and continuing to cook gently over a low–medium heat until it starts to turn brown and smells nutty. Take off the heat and continue to swirl around as the residual heat will continue to turn all the butter brown. Add the lemon juice, then stir in the chives and matcha.

In a large frying pan, heat the coconut oil and sauté the lemon zest over a medium heat for a minute until the aromas are released. Add the prawns and cook for just a couple of minutes, then add the matcha butter.

Meanwhile, whisk the eggs and milk together. Heat a nonstick frying pan (skillet) and add a little butter. Dip the brioche slices one by one in the egg mixture, then add to the pan, cooking for about 3 minutes on each side until golden.

Serve the prawns on top of the eggy brioche and serve with sliced kombu and pea shoots, if using.

SERVES 2

MATCHA SCRAMBLED EGGS
with creamed corn

Matcha works brilliantly as a seasoning; here we've mixed it with some sea salt flakes. Always use a spatula when making scrambled eggs and you will have the perfect soft curds. If cream feels a little too indulgent, swap for crème fraîche (soured cream).

FOR THE CREAMED CORN
25 g (1 oz) unsalted butter
100 g (3½ oz) frozen sweetcorn, defrosted
1 teaspoon paprika
2 tablespoons single (light) cream

FOR THE EGGS
4 eggs
2 tablespoons single cream
10 g (¼ oz) unsalted butter

TO SERVE
¼ teaspoon matcha powder
1 teaspoon sea salt flakes
2 slices of sourdough bread
fresh sweet cicely leaves, to garnish (optional)

Start by making the creamed corn. Place a pan over a medium heat and, when hot, add the butter. Once the butter is melted and beginning to bubble, add the sweetcorn and toss to coat in the butter. Add the paprika and cream and continue to toss for a few minutes, until the sweetcorn is cooked through, all the flavours have combined and the cream is reduced.

For the scrambled eggs, whisk the eggs vigorously with the cream in a bowl. Heat a nonstick pan until extremely hot then add the butter. Allow to melt, then add the whisked egg mixture. Stir with a spatula to make curds until the eggs are almost done. Remove from the heat and the eggs will finish cooking in the residual heat of the pan.

Mix the matcha powder and salt together. Toast the sourdough, then add the creamed corn and scrambled eggs on top. Sprinkle with a little matcha, salt and sweet cicely, if using, to serve.

SOUPS, SIDES & SNACKS

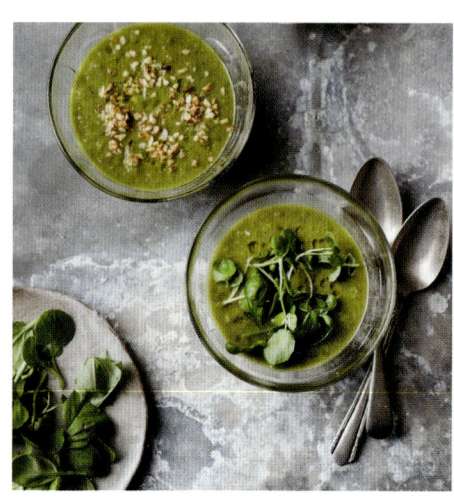

25	**Spiced Watercress & Matcha Soup**
26	**Matcha Mushroom Noodle Soup**
27	**Matcha Buckwheat Broth**
29	**Cauliflower Soup**
31	**Ramen**
32	**Pea, Mint & Matcha Soup**
33	**Matcha & Red Lentil Hummus**
34	**Matcha Salt**
34	**Lemon Matcha Butter**
35	**Matcha Pickles**
36	**Soured Cucumber Salad**
38	**White Asparagus**
39	**Matcha Miso Aubergine**
41	**Baked Matcha Cauliflower**
43	**Cheese & Matcha Scones**

SERVES 4

SPICED WATERCRESS & MATCHA SOUP

The intense, vibrant green of this soup sings its own healthy praises, plus it has flavour to match.

---

1 tablespoon olive oil
1 leek, sliced
2 teaspoons matcha powder
pinch of cayenne pepper
pinch of ground cloves
¼ teaspoon ground ginger
¼ teaspoon ground coriander
¼ teaspoon ground cardamom
½ teaspoon grated nutmeg
350 g (12 oz) spinach
150 g (5½ oz) watercress, plus extra to garnish
½ teaspoon sea salt
good pinch of black pepper
600 ml (20 fl oz) hot vegetable stock (broth)

TO SERVE
handful of hazelnuts, chopped (optional)

Heat the olive oil in a saucepan and add the leek. Sauté over a medium heat for 10 minutes, until soft. Add the matcha powder and all the ground spices, stirring and cooking for another 5 minutes.

Add the spinach, watercress, salt and pepper and stir through, then add the hot stock and stir just until the leaves have wilted. Use a hand-held blender to blitz as soon as possible in order to retain the bright green colour. Garnish with extra watercress and a sprinkling of chopped hazelnuts, if liked.

SERVES 2

MATCHA MUSHROOM NOODLE SOUP

Mushrooms have their own distinctive hint of umami, which forms the basis of this soup in the shiitake dashi, or stock (broth). The matcha adds another layer when you put together the elements for the soup.

---

10 g (⅓ oz) dried shiitake mushrooms
400 ml (14 fl oz) water
200 g (7 oz) udon noodles
2 tablespoons soy sauce
1 tablespoon mirin
1 tablespoon sesame oil
100 g (3½ oz) fresh enoki or shiitake mushrooms
1 teaspoon matcha powder
100 g (3½ oz) baby spinach leaves, shredded

To make the mushroom dashi (stock) for the soup, soak the dried mushrooms in the water overnight.

When you are ready to make the soup, bring the mushroom dashi to the boil in a saucepan, along with the soaked mushrooms. Add the udon noodles, soy sauce and mirin and cook for about 4–5 minutes.

At the same time, heat the sesame oil in a frying pan (skillet) and add the fresh mushrooms. Sprinkle with the matcha powder and cook over a medium–high heat for a couple of minutes. Add the spinach, stir through to wilt slightly, then remove from the heat.

Divide the mushrooms and spinach between 2 bowls and ladle over the noodle broth.

SERVES 2

MATCHA BUCKWHEAT BROTH

Buckwheat is an ancient grain-like seed that is a great gluten-free alternative to wheat. It also comes in noodle form, which would work equally well in this recipe.

- 600 ml (20 fl oz) chicken or vegetable stock (broth)
- 1 lemon grass stalk, bashed
- 100 g (3½ oz) buckwheat
- 1 tablespoon coconut oil
- 100 g (3½ oz) cavolo nero or kale, stalks removed and leaves shredded
- 1 teaspoon grated fresh root ginger
- ½ teaspoon matcha powder
- 2 tablespoons wheat-free tamari soy sauce

Bring the stock to the boil in a saucepan. Add the lemon grass and buckwheat, reduce to a simmer and cook for about 10 minutes, or until the buckwheat is tender.

Meanwhile, heat the coconut oil in a frying pan (skillet) or wok, add the greens, ginger and matcha powder and sauté for about 5 minutes, adding the soy sauce just as the greens become tender.

Remove the lemon grass and divide the broth between two bowls, topping with the ginger matcha greens.

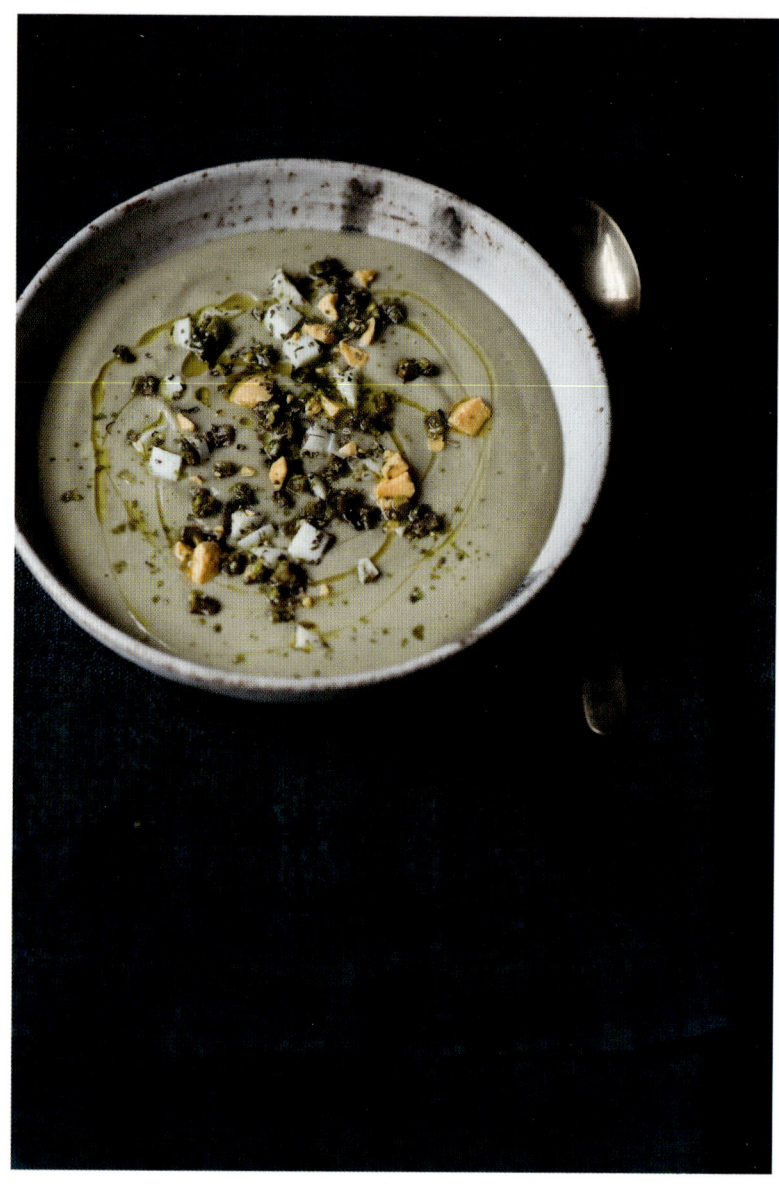

SERVES 4

CAULIFLOWER SOUP
with matcha mimosa

Cauliflower goes well with matcha, but rather than turn this soup a greenish colour, we decided to make a topping with chopped egg and a little matcha powder used as a seasoning.

---

1 large cauliflower
1 tablespoon unsalted butter
¾ teaspoon matcha powder
500 ml (18 fl oz) unsweetened almond milk
250 ml (9 fl oz) chicken stock (broth)
2 eggs
½ celery stick, finely chopped
1 teaspoon dried oregano
sea salt
sesame oil, for drizzling

Cut the cauliflower into small pieces. Heat the butter in a large saucepan, add the cauliflower and a good pinch of salt and sauté over a medium–high heat for a few minutes.

Add half a teaspoon of the matcha powder, then the almond milk and stock. Bring to the boil and simmer for about 10–15 minutes, or until the cauliflower is cooked. Transfer to a blender and whizz until smooth (or use a hand-held blender). Taste for seasoning.

Meanwhile, add the eggs to a pan of boiling water and boil for 8 minutes. Cool them under running water, then peel and chop. Mix together with the chopped celery, the remaining matcha powder, oregano and a little salt.

Ladle the soup into bowls, drizzle with sesame oil and top with the matcha mimosa.

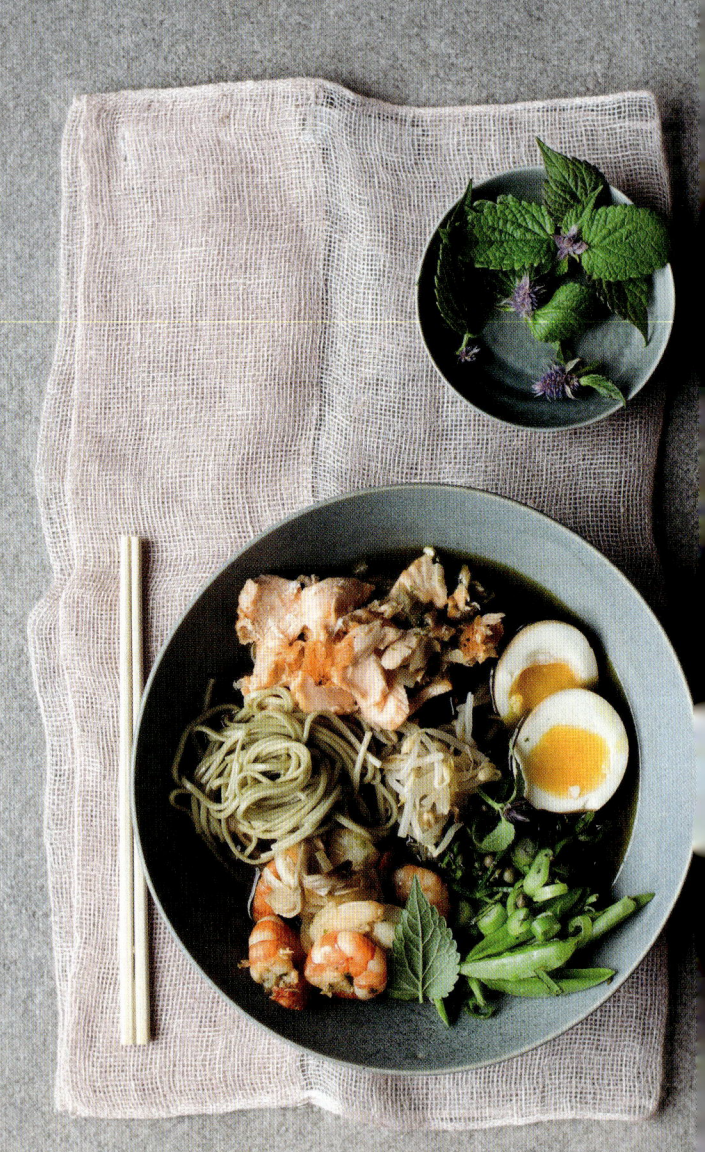

SERVES 2

RAMEN

You can take any of the elements in this dish and combine them however you like, adding different vegetables or proteins that you like, such as pork, chicken or tofu. Matcha noodles are great if you can find them, or just use your favourite type.

---

100 g (3½ oz) matcha noodles (or any soba noodles)
2 eggs
350 ml (12 fl oz) chicken or vegetable stock (broth)
1 teaspoon matcha powder
1 teaspoon green curry paste
4 dried or fresh kaffir lime leaves
1 tablespoon fish sauce
250 ml (9 fl oz) water
100 g (3½ oz) raw king prawns (jumbo shrimp)
200 g (7 oz) flaked poached salmon
50 g (2 oz) mangetout (snow peas), sliced in half
1 spring onion (scallion), sliced
50 g (2 oz) bean sprouts

TO SERVE

anise hyssop leaves or any fresh herb, to serve (optional)

Cook the noodles in boiling water following the packet instructions. Refresh in cold water and drain.

Meanwhile, bring a saucepan of water to the boil, add the eggs and boil for 6 minutes (or longer if you prefer hard-boiled). Cool under running cold water before peeling and slicing into halves. Set aside.

Put the stock into a large pan and stir in the matcha powder, curry paste, lime leaves, fish sauce and water. Bring to a simmer and cook for 15 minutes to infuse the flavours. Add the raw prawns and leave to simmer for another 5 minutes, until they turn pink. Remove from the heat and add the flaked salmon.

Divide the noodles between 2 deep bowls and pour over the broth, dividing the prawns and salmon evenly between the servings. Garnish with the egg halves, mangetout, spring onion, bean sprouts and herb leaves, if using.

SERVES 2

PEA, MINT & MATCHA SOUP

This is such a vibrant soup, perfect for summer when garden peas are at their finest. At other times of year, you can always use frozen peas, still very fresh, as they are frozen as soon as they are picked.

- 80 g (3 oz) chilled butter
- 1 leek, thinly sliced
- 2 garlic cloves, thinly sliced
- 1 medium waxy potato, peeled and diced
- 500 ml (18 fl oz) vegetable stock
- 250 g (8 oz) garden peas
- 2 teaspoons matcha powder, plus extra for dusting
- 15 g mint leaves
- juice of ½ lime
- 2 teaspoons crème fraîche or natural (plain) yogurt
- sea salt

Melt half the butter in a saucepan over a medium heat and fry the leek and garlic until softened. Add the diced potato and cook, stirring, for 2 minutes. Add the stock and a large pinch of salt and bring to a simmer.

Once the potatoes are cooked and offer little resistance to a knife, add the peas and matcha powder, bring back to a simmer and cook for another 2–3 minutes. Remove the pan from the heat, add the mint, reserving a few leaves to garnish, and set aside to infuse for another couple of minutes.

Reserve 2 ladles of cooking liquid, then blend the mixture using a hand-held blender. Dice the remaining chilled butter and whisk into the blended soup one at a time. If the mixture appears too thick – more like a purée than a soup – add some of the reserved liquid until the desired consistency has been reached.

Pass the blended soup though a fine sieve and stir in the lime juice. Garnish with a teaspoon of crème fraîche or yogurt and a sprig of mint.

SERVES 4

MATCHA & RED LENTIL HUMMUS

Hummus is such a great healthy snack; here we've used lentils instead of chickpeas, although you can easily swap them. If using chickpeas, it's a good idea to add a little water and olive oil to the mix.

---

100 g (3½ oz) dried red lentils, rinsed and drained
1 garlic clove, crushed
juice of ½ lemon, or to taste
1 tablespoon tahini
¼ teaspoon sea salt
¼ teaspoon matcha powder

Add the red lentils to a saucepan, along with enough water to cover by 1 cm (½ in).

Bring to the boil, then reduce the heat and simmer for about 15 minutes, or until cooked and soft. Drain and set aside to cool.

Add the cooled lentils to a food processor or blender along with the remaining ingredients and blend to a soft, hummus-like consistency.

Taste and adjust the seasoning, adding more lemon juice if needed.

MAKES 1½ TABLESPOONS

MATCHA SALT

Matcha works well when you think of it as a seasoning, adding just that last hint or layer of flavour as a finishing touch to a dish. This matcha salt is delicious with eggs (see page 23), and to season fish or meat.

---

1 tablespoon sea salt flakes
½ teaspoon matcha powder

Combine the salt and matcha. Voilà.

MAKES ABOUT 125 G (4½ OZ)

LEMON MATCHA BUTTER

Having a flavoured butter on hand means that you can add amazing flavour to the simplest of dishes. This lemon matcha butter is particularly good with any pan-fried or baked fish, from lemon sole to cod (or anything that looks good that day at the fishmonger). Cook your fish as normal and add a disc of flavoured butter at the end, allowing it to melt in the pan and spooning the melted butter over the fish as it rests.

---

125 g (4½ oz) butter
zest of 1 lemon
1 tablespoon matcha powder

Once the butter is soft enough beat the lemon zest and matcha into it.

Shape into a log and chill. Once cold, wrap the log in clingfilm (plastic wrap), knotting the ends, so that you can unwrap and slice off discs of butter as you need them.

SERVES 6

MATCHA PICKLES

Pickling and fermenting have come back into fashion, not least because these methods of preserving food are very healthy. Pickles are a really good way to add a burst of flavour to a simple dish, such as a sandwich, spring rolls (see page 55), fish or a burger (see page 59).

FOR THE PICKLED EGGS
6 eggs
250 ml (9 fl oz) cider vinegar
150 ml (5 fl oz) water
50 g (2 oz) coconut sugar
1 teaspoon sea salt
1 teaspoon fennel seeds
1 teaspoon mustards seeds
3 bay leaves
1 whole green chilli
1 tablespoon matcha powder

FOR THE PICKLED
 VEGETABLES
1 large carrot, cut into batons
1 large cucumber, halved lengthways, deseeded and cut into batons
½ medium cauliflower, cut into small florets
¼ onion, sliced
250 ml (9 fl oz) brown rice vinegar
150 ml (5 fl oz) water
50 g (2 oz) coconut sugar
1 teaspoon sea salt
1 teaspoon matcha powder

Start by sterilizing the pickling jars you are going to use by pouring boiling-hot water over them and leaving them for several minutes. Pour the water out and leave them to air-dry.

To make the pickled eggs, bring a pan of water to the boil. Add the eggs and boil for 6 minutes, then run under cold water before peeling and placing in a sterilized jar. Meanwhile, put all the remaining egg ingredients into a pan, bring to the boil and simmer for a couple of minutes.

Allow the pickling liquor to cool a little, then pour over the eggs. Seal and when cool, transfer to the refrigerator, where they will keep for up to 4 weeks.

To make the pickled vegetables, place the prepared vegetables in a sterilized jar. Make the pickling liquor as above and pour over.

SERVES 4

SOURED CUCUMBER SALAD
with goats' curd

This is delicious as part of a summer barbecue or gathering. You can make a big batch of the cucumbers as they'll keep for up to a month: just double or triple the quantities.

FOR THE CUCUMBERS

200 ml (7 fl oz) white wine vinegar
2 tablespoons caster (superfine) sugar
1 teaspoon pink peppercorns
1 tablespoon mustard seeds
2 baby cucumbers, chopped into wedges
1 teaspoon sea salt
50 g (2 oz) dill
120 g (4 oz) goats' curd

TO SERVE

4 slices wholemeal bread, toasted
½ teaspoon Matcha Salt (see page 34)
20 g (¾ oz) dill

Heat the vinegar, sugar, peppercorns and mustard seeds in a saucepan, stirring until the sugar has dissolved. Set aside to cool.

Place the cucumber wedges in a colander and toss with the salt. Leave to stand for 15 minutes before transferring to a sterilized jar (see page 35) along with the dill. Pour over the cooled vinegar and sugar solution and seal with an airtight lid. The cucumbers will be sour enough to eat a day later, but will keep up to a month in the refrigerator, becoming more sour over time.

Spread the curd on a serving plate and arrange the cucumber wedges on top. Serve with the toast and finish by sprinkling over the matcha salt, dill and a little pickling liquor.

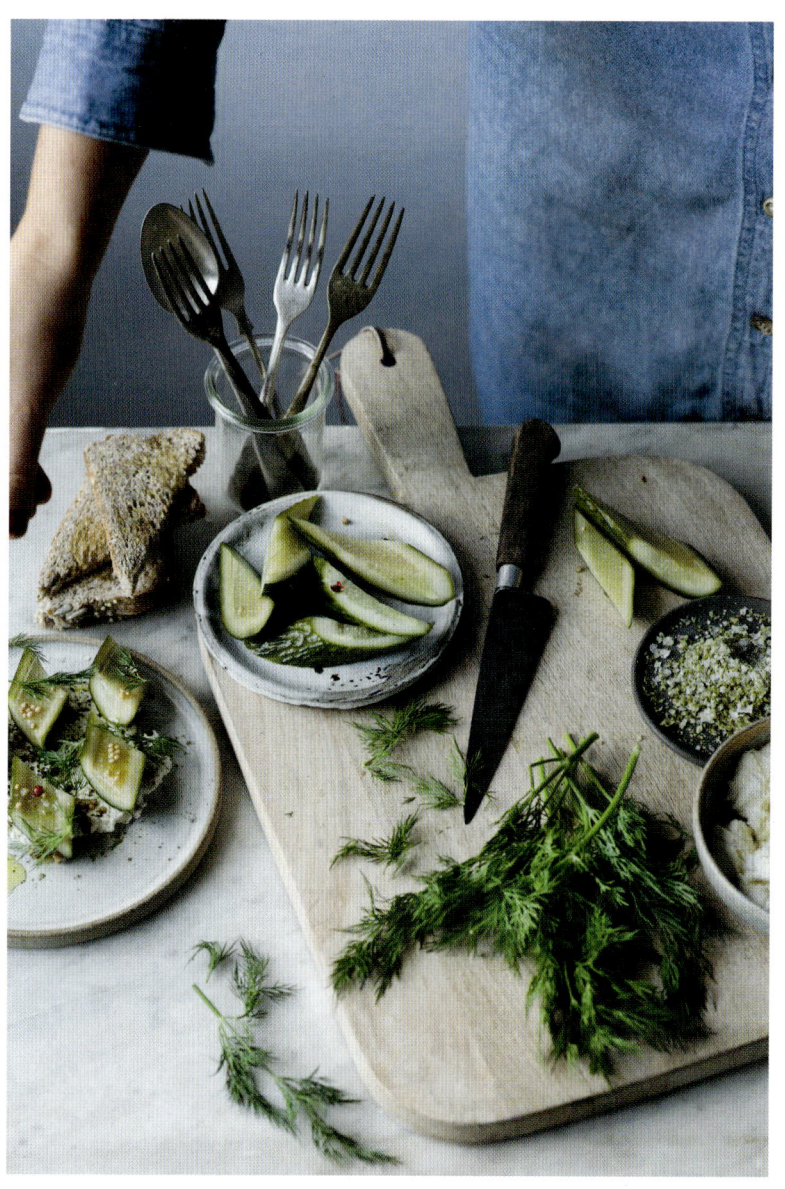

SERVES 4

WHITE ASPARAGUS
with matcha vinaigrette & quail eggs

White asparagus is only in season for a short time, but is absolutely delicious if you come across it. Although thicker than green asparagus, it is usually very tender and sweet.

½ garlic clove, finely grated
1 teaspoon Dijon mustard
½ teaspoon honey
2 tablespoons white wine vinegar
1 teaspoon matcha powder
3 tablespoons olive oil
8 quail eggs
8–12 white asparagus spears, or use 16–20 green asparagus spears

TO SERVE
4 teaspoons ground flaxseed (optional)
sea salt and ground black pepper

Mix together the garlic, mustard, honey, vinegar and matcha powder in a bowl. Add the oil gradually, whisking hard so that you end up with a creamy vinaigrette.

Bring a saucepan of water to the boil. Lower the quail eggs in and cook for 2½ minutes. Remove from the water and place straight into a bowl of cold water before peeling.

Snap off and discard the tough ends of the asparagus, then shave the spears using a peeler so you end up with very thin slices – don't worry about making them overly neat. Divide the asparagus shavings between 4 plates so it covers the surface of each one.

Cut the quail eggs in half and lay 4 halves randomly on each plate. Spoon over the creamy matcha vinaigrette and dust with ground flaxseed, if using. Season with salt and pepper and serve.

SERVES 2

MATCHA MISO AUBERGINE

Sweet miso aubergine is so easy and so delicious. Matcha makes a good addition to the classic recipe as it goes well with ginger and soy. Here we've used furikake – a brilliant Japanese seasoning made from black and white sesame seeds and seaweed flakes – to sprinkle over the roasted aubergines. It's available in many supermarkets and health food stores, but if you can't find it, sesame seeds work can be used instead.

---

2 aubergines (eggplant)
1 heaped tablespoon white miso paste
1 tablespoon honey
1 tablespoon soy sauce
1 teaspoon toasted sesame oil
1 teaspoon grated fresh root ginger
1 teaspoon matcha powder
3 spring onions (scallions), shredded
2 teaspoons furikake or sesame seeds

Preheat the oven to 180°C (350°F), Gas Mark 4.

Slice the aubergines in half lengthways and score the flesh in a diamond pattern. Place the aubergine halves, scored-side up, on a baking tray.

Mix the miso, honey, soy sauce, sesame oil, ginger and matcha powder together, adding just a little water to loosen to a smooth paste. Brush this over the aubergines.

Roast in the oven for about 20 minutes, or until golden in colour and soft all the way through. Serve scattered with the shredded spring onions and sprinkle over the furikake (or sesame seeds).

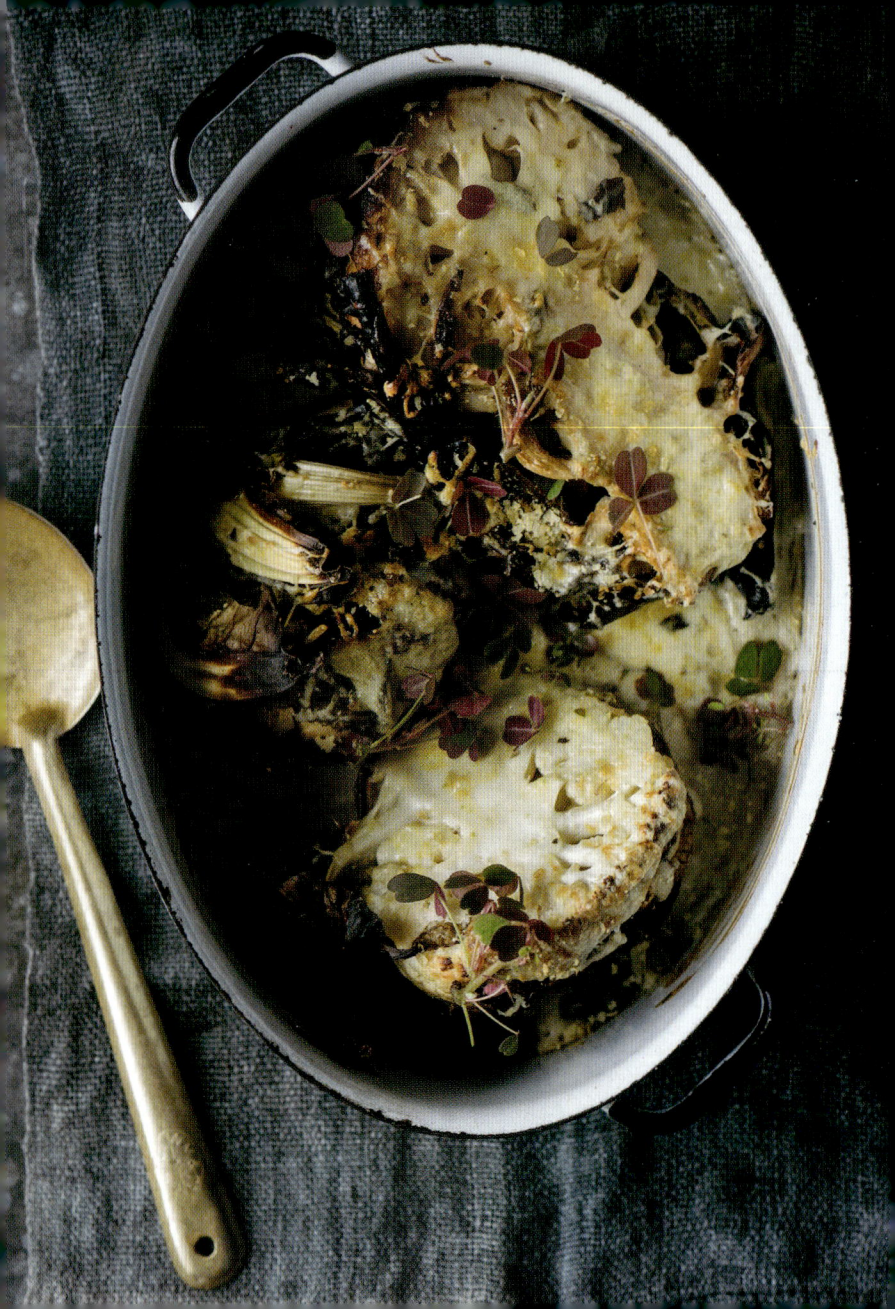

SERVES 4

BAKED MATCHA CAULIFLOWER

You can make this vegan by leaving out the Cheddar cheese at the end, although it does add wonderful colour and a bit of extra lusciousness. The white miso, while optional, will add a boost of umami flavour.

---

1 medium whole cauliflower
1½ tablespoons coconut oil
1 onion, quartered
2 garlic cloves, halved
400 ml (14 fl oz) oat milk
2 teaspoons matcha powder
225 g (8 oz) cashew nuts, soaked overnight or for at least 4 hours
50 g (2 oz) brewer's yeast or nutritional yeast
1 teaspoon white miso (optional)
generous handful of grated mild Cheddar cheese (optional)
sea salt and ground black pepper
red sorrel, to garnish (optional)

Preheat the oven to 220°C (425°F), Gas Mark 7.

Discard the largest outer leaves from the cauliflower, then cut into quarters. Bring a deep saucepan of salted water to the boil. Add the cauliflower and boil for 10 minutes, until tender, then transfer to a baking tray.

Meanwhile, melt the coconut oil in a saucepan, and fry the onion and garlic over a medium heat until slightly transparent. Add the oat milk and matcha powder and bring to the boil. Once boiled, pour this mixture into a blender and add the drained cashew nuts, yeast and white miso, if using. Blend on a high speed for 2 minutes, until you have a very smooth, luxurious sauce. Season to taste.

Pour the sauce all over the cauliflower. Sprinkle the grated Cheddar, if using, over the top, then roast in the oven for 20 minutes. Garnish with red sorrel, if using.

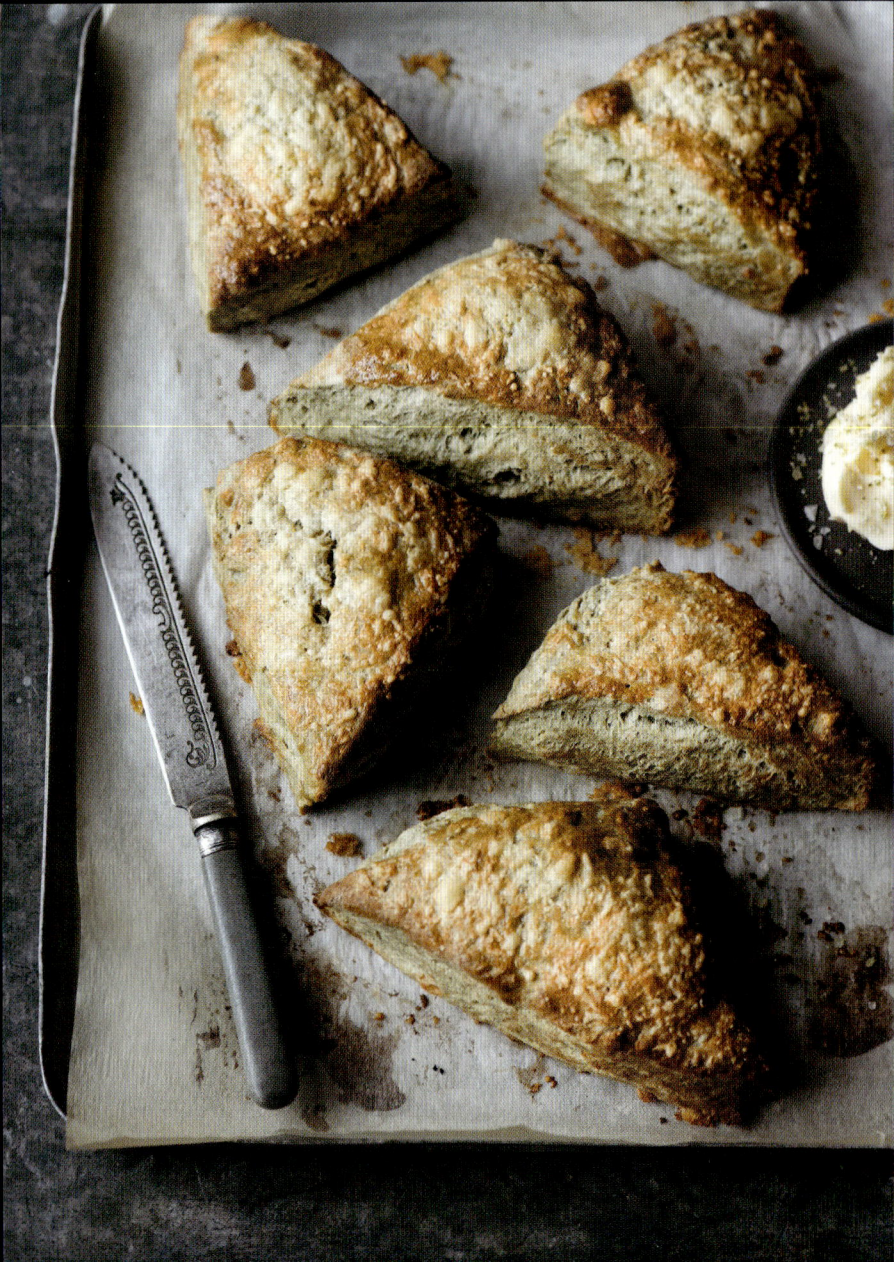

MAKES ABOUT 6 LARGE SCONES

CHEESE & MATCHA SCONES

These cheesy scones are the perfect showcase for a spot of matcha-inspired baking.

---

450 g (14½ oz) self-raising flour, plus extra for dusting
1 teaspoon sea salt
1 tablespoon matcha powder
100 g (3½ oz) chilled unsalted butter, cut into small cubes
250 g (8 oz) mature Cheddar cheese, finely grated
120 ml (4 fl oz) cold milk or buttermilk
120 ml (4 fl oz) cold water
1 egg, beaten with a splash of milk

Preheat the oven to 220°C (425°F), Gas Mark 7.

Put the flour, salt and matcha powder into a large bowl and mix together until well combined. Add the butter and rub it into the flour with your fingertips until it looks grainy.

Add 225 g (7½ oz) of the cheese and stir to combine. Mix in the milk and water, until the dough just comes away from the side of the bowl. Transfer to a lightly floured surface and flatten the dough into a rectangle about 2.5 cm (1 in) thick. Using a sharp knife, cut into 6 large triangles. Gently push any offcuts together to cut more shapes.

Transfer the dough to a baking tray lined with baking paper (parchment) and brush with the egg and milk mixture. Sprinkle the remaining cheese over the tops and bake for about 12 minutes, or until golden. Transfer to a wire rack to cool before serving.

MAIN DISHES

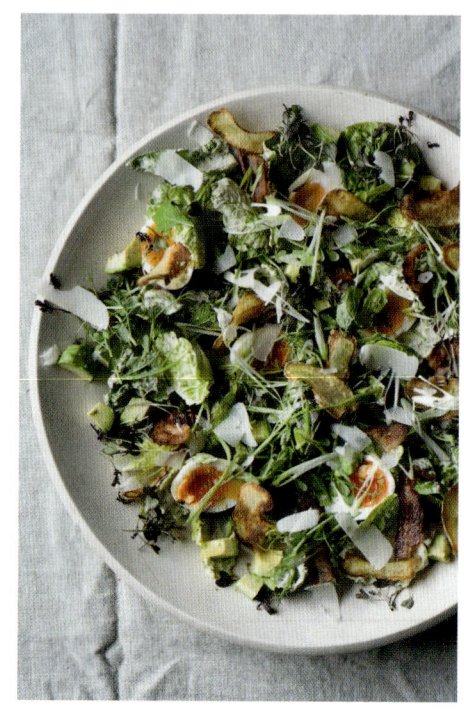

45	**Bacon, Lettuce & Matcha Salad**
47	**Matcha Mushroom Spelt Risotto**
48	**Matcha Noodles**
50	**Trout**
52	**Sole**
53	**Salmon**
55	**Summer Rolls**
56	**Matcha Poached Chicken**
59	**Matcha Burger**

SERVES 4

BACON, LETTUCE & MATCHA SALAD

This salad is really quick and open to variation – you could include chicken, or swap the bacon for tofu to make a vegetarian option.

---

1 teaspoon unsalted butter
4 slices of streaky bacon, cut into 2.5 cm (1 in) slices
2 baby gem lettuces, leaves separated
1 ripe avocado, peeled, stoned and cut into small pieces
3 hard-boiled eggs, halved

FOR THE DRESSING
100 g (3½ oz) Greek yogurt
1 teaspoon matcha poweder
zest and juice of ½ lime
1 teaspoon ume shiso seasoning or cider vinegar

FOR THE MATCHA CRISPS
1 potato
2 tablespoons olive oil
1 teaspoon Matcha Salt (see page 34)

TO SERVE
Parmesan shavings
a handful of pea shoots
2 spring onions (scallions), sliced

First make the lime dressing. Combine all the ingredients in a bowl, adjusting the flavour to taste. Set aside.

To make the matcha crisps, slice the potato as thinly as possible with a mandolin or sharp knife. Pat dry with kitchen paper (paper towel), then toss in the olive oil and matcha salt. Tip on to a baking tray and bake for 2 hours, turning over halfway through, until golden. Remove from the oven and rest for 10 minutes to continue crisping up.

In the meantime, heat a frying pan (skillet) and melt the butter. Add the bacon and cook until crisp.

Put the lettuce leaves into a large mixing bowl and gently combine with the yogurt dressing until evenly coated. Place in a serving dish, then add the avocado, bacon, eggs, and matcha crisps.

To serve, sprinkle over the Parmesan, pea shoots and spring onions.

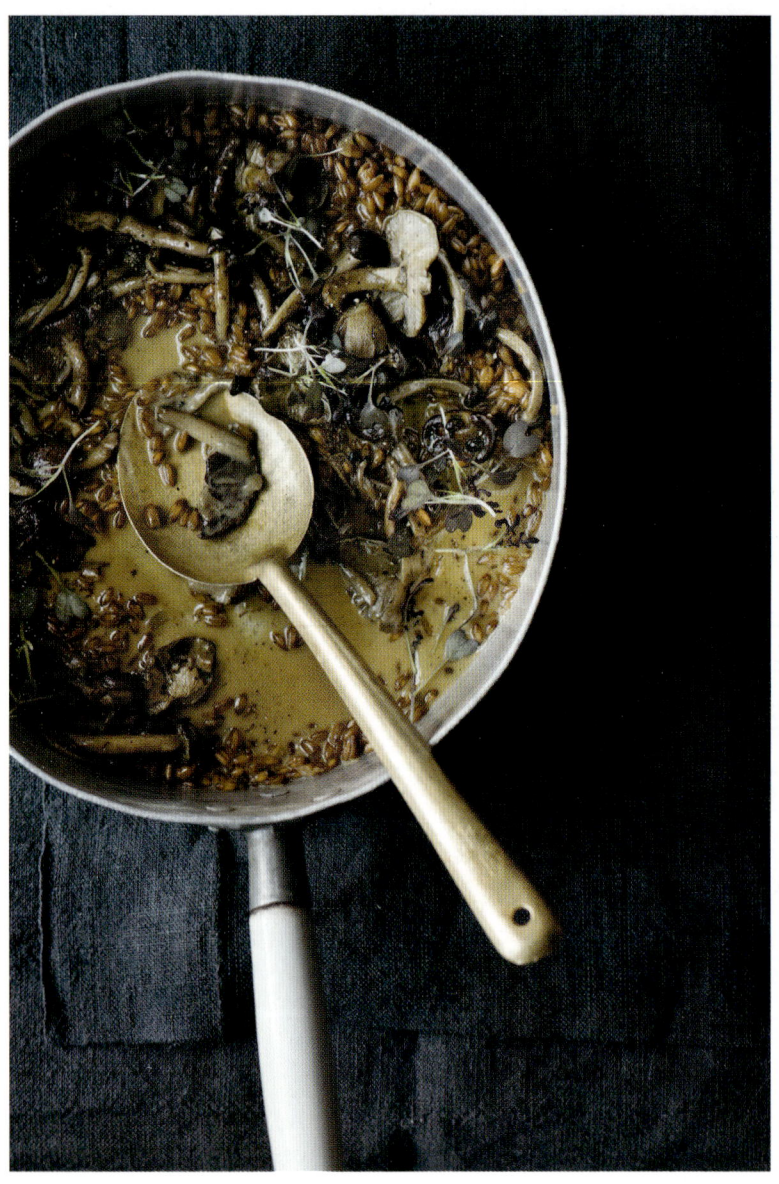

SERVES 2

MATCHA MUSHROOM SPELT RISOTTO

Mushrooms go really well with matcha, especially when helped along with a little butter, as in this recipe. Shiitake and shimejii mushrooms are used here, but this risotto would work equally well with chestnut (cremini) mushrooms.

---

160 g (5¾ oz) spelt grains, soaked overnight, rinsed and drained
1 tablespoon olive oil
1 small onion, finely chopped
300 ml (10 fl oz) hot vegetable or chicken stock (broth)
1 tablespoon unsalted butter
100 g (3½ oz) mixed shimejii and shiitake mushrooms, cleaned
½ teaspoon matcha powder
1 tablespoon yeast flakes or grated Parmesan cheese
sea salt
red lace mustard leaves, to garnish (optional)

Add the spelt grains to a saucepan and cover well with water. Bring to the boil, then simmer for 20 minutes. Drain, rinse and set aside.

Place the olive oil in a large saucepan over a medium heat and sauté the onion for about 10 minutes. Add the spelt, stirring to coat all the grains in the oil.

Ladle half the hot stock into the grains, bring to the boil, then reduce to a gentle simmer and cook for about 10 minutes, stirring occasionally. Add more stock as needed to cook the spelt and create a risotto-like texture.

Meanwhile, melt the butter in a separate pan and sauté the mushrooms with the matcha powder and a little sea salt.

Either stir the mushrooms through the cooked spelt or pile the mushrooms on top of it in bowls. Sprinkle with yeast flakes or grated Parmesan, and garnish with red lace mustard leaves, if using.

SERVES 2

MATCHA NOODLES
with tofu

Like matcha, ingredients such as kombu seaweed and furikake are now more easily available in supermarkets, Asian stores and online. For a simpler version of the broth in this recipe, you can use miso instead of the kombu and lemon grass, and add the matcha, mirin and tamari as below.

---

1 sheet of kombu
400 ml (14 fl oz) vegetable stock (broth)
1 lemon grass stalk, bashed
4–6 dried shiitake mushrooms
2 teaspoons matcha powder
1 tablespoon mirin
2 tablespoons tamari
200 g (7 oz) matcha noodles
200 g (7 oz) firm tofu, cut into cubes
2 teaspoons nori flakes
1 teaspoon sesame seeds
1 tablespoon sesame oil
1 pak choi, roughly chopped
squeeze of lime juice
baby salad leaves, to garnish (optional)

To make the dashi broth, put the kombu into a saucepan with the hot vegetable stock, lemon grass, shiitake mushrooms and matcha powder. Bring to the boil and simmer for 20 minutes. Discard the kombu and lemon grass, then add the mirin and tamari.

Bring a large saucepan of water to the boil, add the noodles and simmer for about 6 minutes, or according to the packet instructions, until cooked. Drain, then refresh with cold water before adding to the broth.

Put the tofu into a bowl, sprinkle over the nori flakes and sesame seeds and toss to mix thoroughly.

Heat the sesame oil in a pan and sauté the pak choi over a medium heat for a couple of minutes.

To assemble, divide the broth and noodles between bowls and top with the tofu and pak choi. Squeeze over the lime juice and garnish with baby salad leaves, if using.

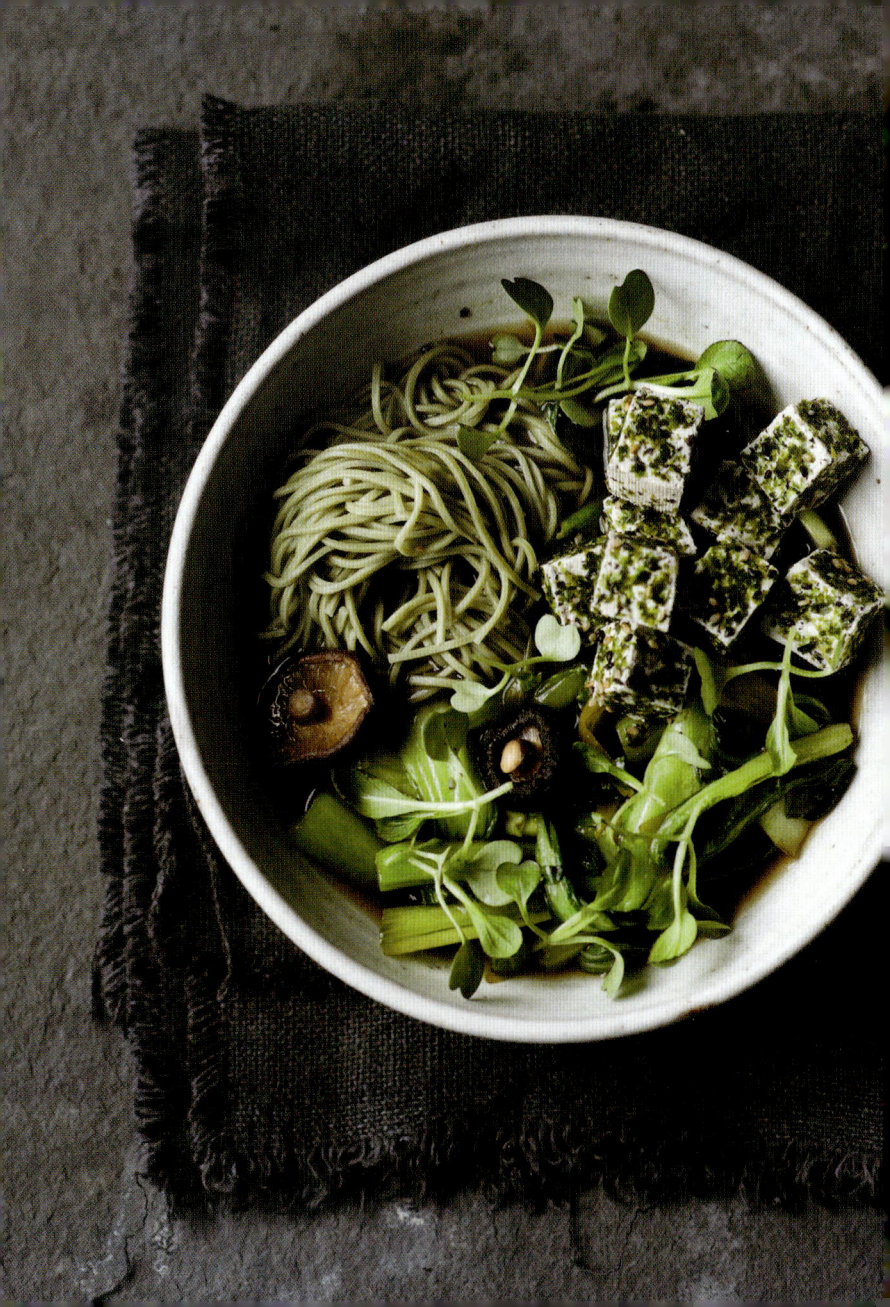

SERVES 2

TROUT
with matcha pistachio crumb

Matcha goes brilliantly with lots of nuts, including hazelnut, almond and the pistachio used here. With this pistachio crumb the colours combine to create a vibrant green crunch that is perfect for fish. If trout isn't in season, the crumb is also delicious with salmon, cod or hake.

---

25 g (1 oz) raw unsalted pistachios
1 teaspoon matcha powder
1 tablespoon breadcrumbs
1 tablespoon olive oil
1 lime, zested then sliced
1 large or 2 small whole rainbow trout, gutted and cleaned (ask your fishmonger to do this)
small handful of soft herbs, such as parsley, chives or coriander (cilantro)
sea salt and ground black pepper

TO SERVE (OPTIONAL)
75 g (3 oz) mixed salad leaves
100 g (3½ oz) heritage tomatoes, thickly sliced
extra virgin olive oil

Preheat the oven to 200°C (400°F), Gas Mark 6 and line a baking tray with baking paper (parchment).

Put the pistachios, matcha powder and breadcrumbs into a food processor and blitz for about 10 seconds, until the pistachios are crumb-like, but not too fine. Mix with the olive oil and lime zest.

Put the trout on the prepared baking tray. With a sharp knife, make 3 diagonal slits along the top of the fish. Season generously and stuff the cavity with any herbs you wish, plus the lime slices.

Press the matcha pistachio crumb all over the top of the trout, reserving some for the salad, if making. Bake in the oven for 8–10 minutes, until the fish is opaque in the middle.

Serve with a tomato salad, if liked. Arrange the salad leaves and sliced tomatoes in a bowl, scatter over the reserved pistachio crumb and drizzle with extra virgin olive oil.

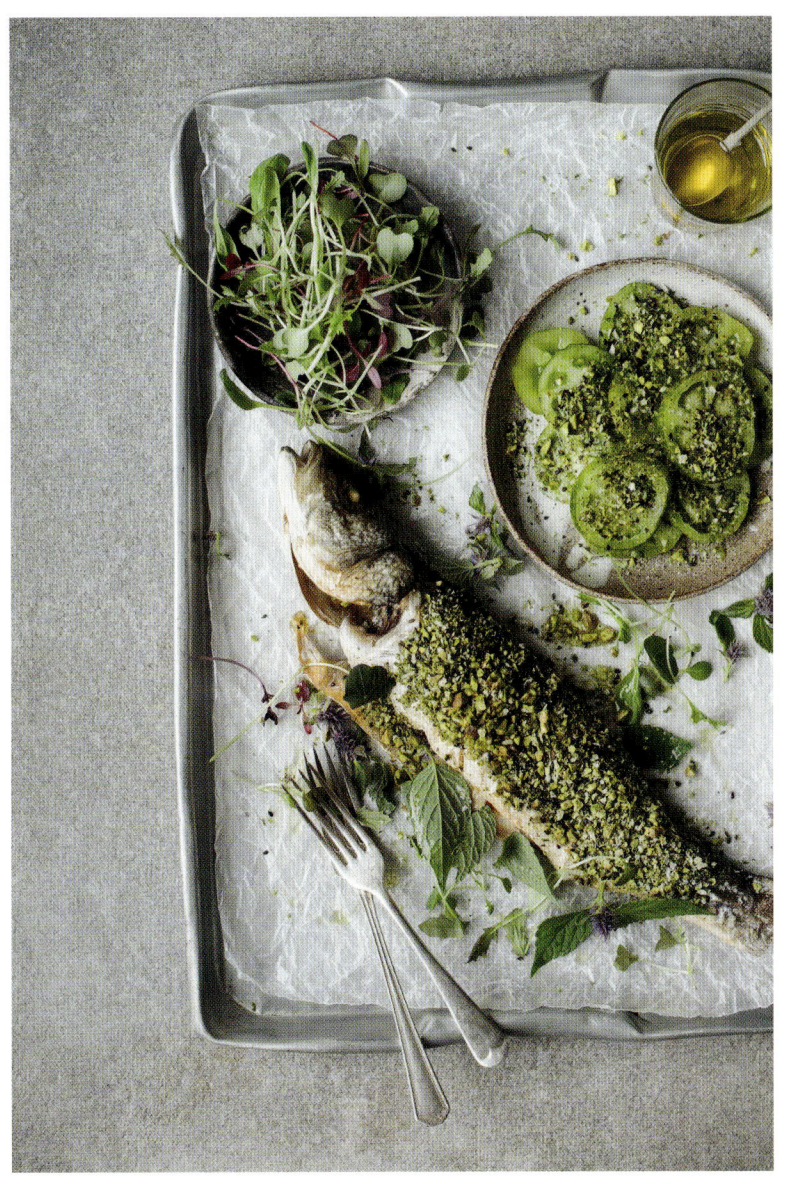

SERVES 2 TO SHARE

SOLE
with matcha beurre blanc & greens

The beurre blanc included here is the perfect way to marry matcha with any white-fleshed fish, such as Dover or lemon sole, but you could use cod, sea bass or any sustainable white fish.

---

1 tablespoon vegetable oil
1 Dover or lemon sole, skinned and trimmed but kept whole
100 g (3½ oz) curly kale, thickly sliced
100 g (3½ oz) cavolo nero, thickly sliced

FOR THE MATCHA BEURRE BLANC
½ garlic clove, sliced
1 shallot, thinly sliced
1 lemon grass stalk, crushed
2.5 cm (1 in) fresh root ginger, peeled and sliced
200 ml (7 fl oz) white wine
60 ml (2½ fl oz) white wine vinegar
1 teaspoon matcha powder
350g (12 oz) chilled butter, diced
squeeze of lemon juice
sea salt

For the matcha beurre blanc, put the garlic, shallot, lemon grass, ginger, wine, vinegar and matcha into a saucepan and bring to the boil. Simmer until the liquid has reduced down by two-thirds.

Remove the lemon grass and reduce the heat to low, then add the chilled butter one piece at a time, making sure each addition has been fully incorporated before adding the next. Strain out the remaining ingredients and you should be left with a thickened, glossy liquid. Add a squeeze of lemon juice and season to taste. Keep the sauce somewhere warm to stop the butter solidifying.

Heat the vegetable oil in a large frying pan (skillet) over a medium heat. When hot, add the sole, skin-side down. Leave for 3–4 minutes, depending on size, until golden, then turn over and cook for another 2–3 minutes.

While the sole is cooking, steam the greens until just cooked, about 3–4 minutes.

Make a bed of the greens on a large plate and place the sole in the middle. Coat the fish in the beurre blanc, making sure the greens get a liberal coating too.

SERVES 2

SALMON
with almond butter matcha crumb

This is a brilliant way to dress up a simple weekday supper. Like nuts, seeds take on the flavour of matcha really well, as they do the mustard and lime.

---

2 thick salmon fillets, about 130 g (4½ oz) each
3 teaspoons wholegrain mustard
2 tablespoons coarse almond butter
30g (1 oz) pumpkin seeds, lightly crushed
zest of 1 lime
⅔ teaspoon matcha powder
1 teaspoon olive oil
1 teaspoon honey
1 tablespoon vegetable oil
sea salt and ground black pepper
lime juice, to serve

Preheat the oven to 240°C (475°F), Gas Mark 9.

Season both sides of the salmon fillets with a light sprinkling of sea salt and set aside.

In the meantime, put 1 teaspoon of the wholegrain mustard into a bowl with the almond butter, pumpkin seeds, lime zest, matcha, olive oil and honey and mix thoroughly to make the crumb. Season with light pinch of salt and a generous amount of pepper.

Pat the salmon fillets dry, then spread the flesh side with the remaining mustard. Spread the crumb evenly on top.

Heat the vegetable oil in an ovenproof frying pan (skillet) over a medium–high heat. Add the salmon fillets, skin-side down, pressing them lightly until they have relaxed and stopped tensing. Transfer to the oven and cook for 4–5 minutes, until the green of the crumb is slightly browned and the fish is medium-rare.

Squeeze lime juice over the salmon before serving.

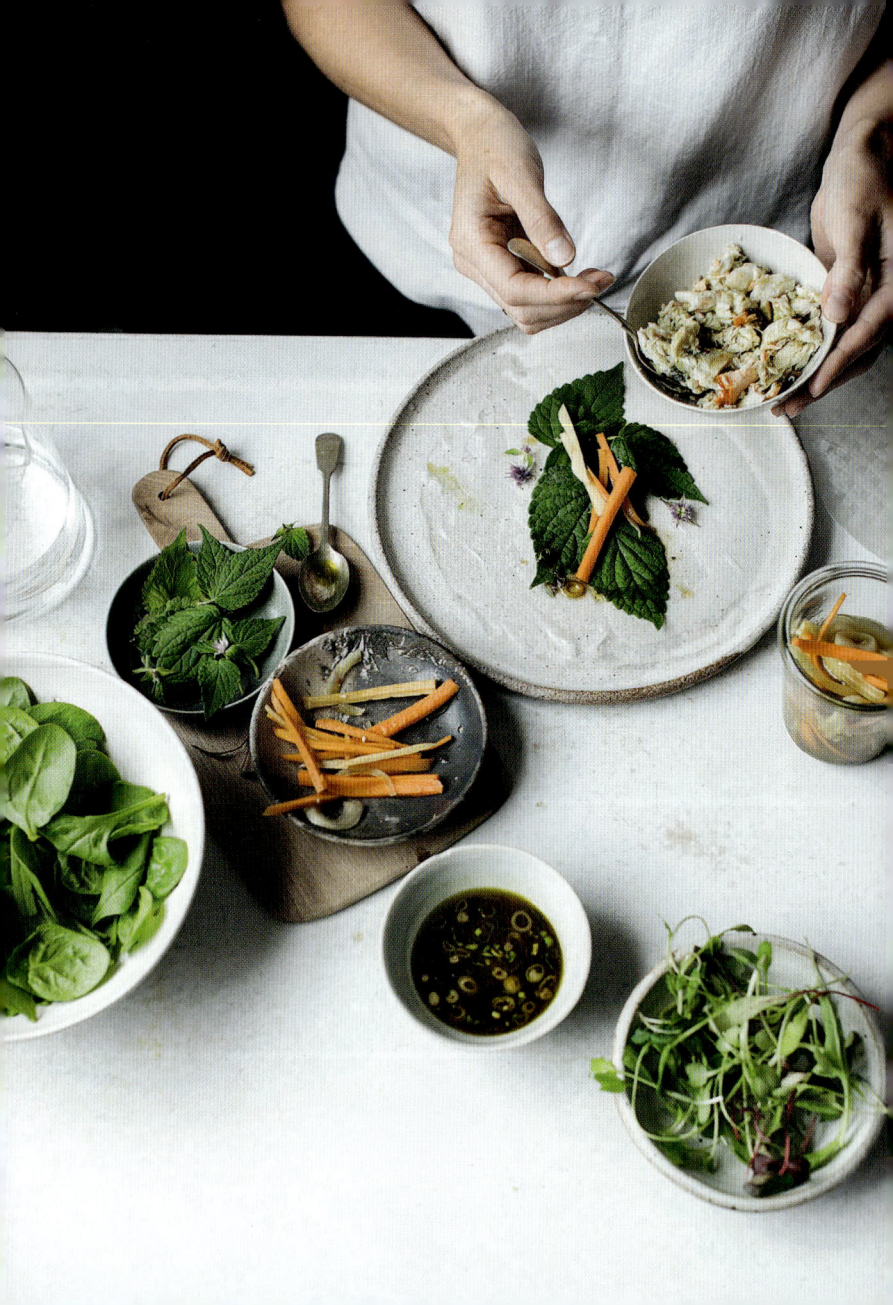

MAKES 8 ROLLS

SUMMER ROLLS
with matcha dipping sauce

Summer rolls, also called 'fresh spring rolls', are a traditional Vietnamese dish made with rice wrappers, raw vegetables and aromatic leaves. The filling often contains prawns, although here we've used lightly steamed fish. Using lettuce or a leaf to line the wrapper before adding your filling adds a delicious extra layer; we've used anise hyssop, but iceberg lettuce works really well too. In this recipe matcha features both in the pickled vegetables and the dipping sauce.

---

8 rice paper wrappers
large handful of anise hyssop leaves (or use 4 iceberg lettuce leaves, halved)
80 g (3 oz) matcha pickled vegetables (see page 35)
200 g (7 oz) steamed salmon or sea bass, flaked
40 g (1½ oz) baby leaf spinach
40 g (1½ oz) coriander (cilantro) leaves

FOR THE DIPPING SAUCE
1 tablespoon coconut sugar
2 tablespoons lime juice
1 tablespoon fish sauce
½ teaspoon matcha powder
1 garlic clove, crushed
1 green chilli, thinly sliced
1 spring onion (scallion), thinly sliced

Fill a large bowl with warm water. Working in batches, soak 2 rice paper wrappers until softened, about 2 minutes. Remove the wrappers from the water and arrange in single layer on your work surface.

Place a few anise hyssop leaves or half an iceberg leaf in the middle of each wrapper. Place a few strips of pickled vegetables in the middle, then a spoonful of steamed fish, then another few strips of pickled vegetables. Add a drizzle of the pickling liquid for flavour and top with a few baby spinach and coriander leaves.

Fold one edge of each wrapper over the filling. Fold in the ends, then roll up tightly, enclosing the filling. Transfer to a serving plate and repeat with remaining wrappers and filling.

To make the dipping sauce, whisk the sugar, lime juice and fish sauce together until dissolved, then whisk in the matcha powder before adding all the other ingredients. Serve in a bowl alongside the summer rolls.

SERVES 2

MATCHA POACHED CHICKEN

The lemon grass in this recipe goes very well with matcha, while poaching the chicken makes it very tender. If you want to be even healthier, replace the new potatoes with another green vegetable.

---

10 g (⅓ oz) unsalted butter
2 teaspoons matcha powder
1 tablespoon nori flakes
2 lemon grass stalks, bashed
400 ml (14 fl oz) chicken stock (broth)
4 chicken thighs
100 g (3½ oz) new potatoes, washed and halved if large
10 g (⅓ oz) lemon matcha butter (see page 34)
200 g (7 oz) asparagus, woody ends snapped off
100 g (3½ oz) baby leeks

Melt the unsalted butter in a heavy-based saucepan over a medium heat and stir in the matcha powder, nori flakes and lemon grass. Pour in the chicken stock and bring to the boil.

Add the chicken thighs, reduce to a simmer and poach for about 15 minutes. Remove the chicken from the poaching liquid and set aside to rest. Return the pan to a high heat and reduce the poaching liquid by half.

Meanwhile, cook the new potatoes in a separate pan of boiling water until tender when pierced with a knife. Drain and set aside.

Melt the lemon matcha butter in a frying pan (skillet) over a medium heat, then add the asparagus and baby leeks. Sauté until tender, about 8 minutes. Remove the vegetables, then place the poached chicken thighs skin-side down in the hot pan to crisp the skin.

Serve the chicken with the potatoes and vegetables, with the reduced poaching liquid drizzled over the top.

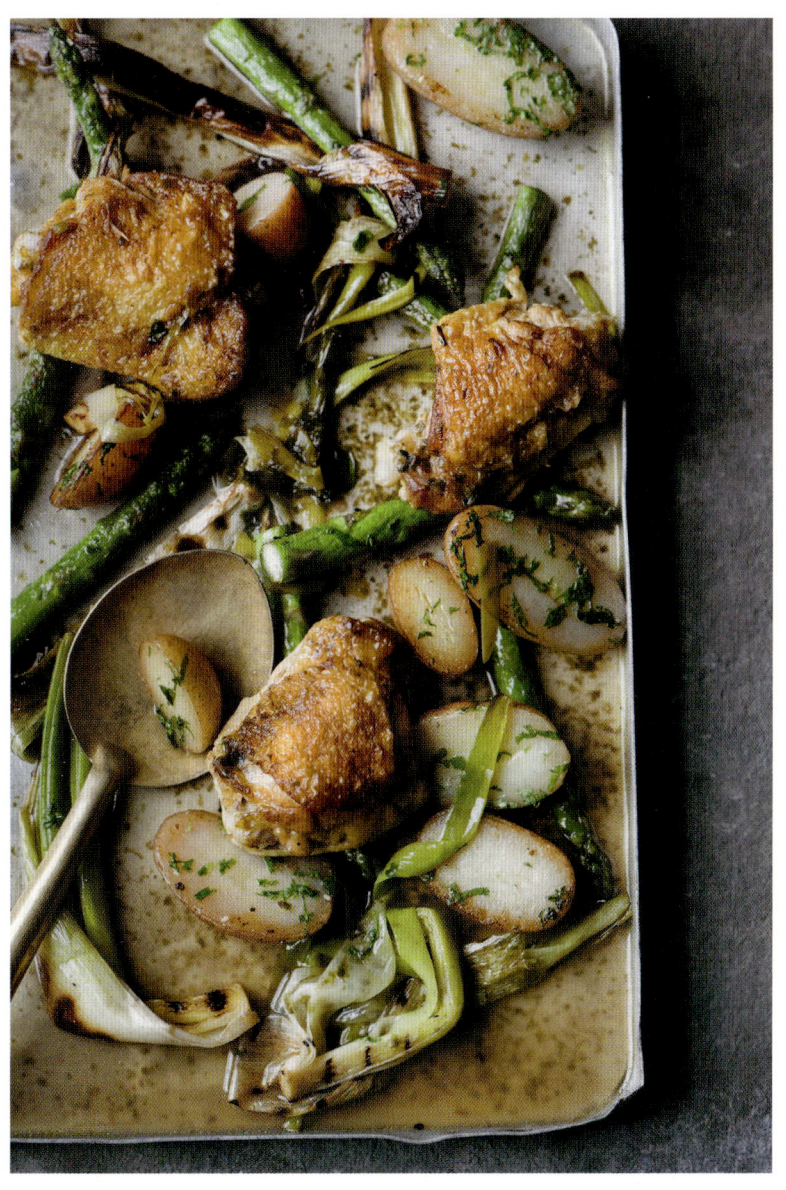

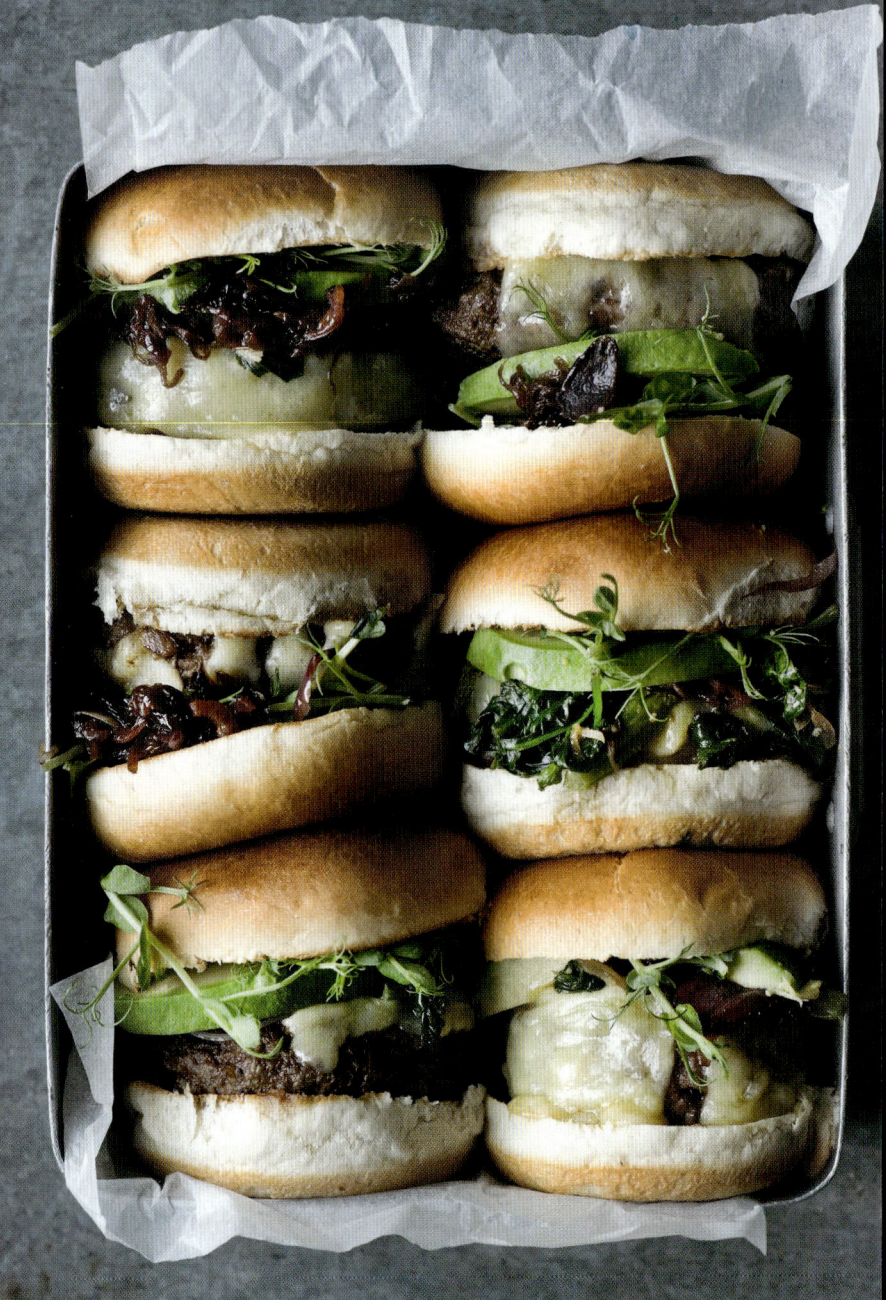

SERVES 4

MATCHA BURGER

Burgers get a bad rap for being unhealthy, but when you make your own, you know exactly what you are putting in, and can choose good-quality, lean meat. While the Cheddar and brioche bun definitely make this a bit of treat, the burger itself is made from simple ingredients.

---

1 onion, finely chopped
1 teaspoon olive oil, plus extra for frying
2 teaspoons matcha powder
400 g (14 oz) minced (ground) beef
1 egg
1 tablespoon Dijon mustard
1 tablespoon Worcestershire sauce
pinch of sea salt

FOR THE ONION JAM
30 g (1 oz) butter
220 g (8 oz) red onion, sliced
1 tablespoon balsamic vinegar

TO SERVE
4 slices of Cheddar cheese (optional)
4 brioche buns, halved and lightly toasted
10 g (⅓ oz) unsalted butter
80 g (2¾ oz) baby spinach
1 avocado, peeled, stoned and sliced
pea shoots or salad leaves

First make the onion jam. Heat a saucepan and melt the butter. Add the onion and a splash of balsamic vinegar. Cook over a low heat for 1½ hours, until the onions are very soft and jam-like.

Sauté the onion in a teaspoon of olive oil for about 10 minutes over a low–medium heat, until soft and translucent, stirring in the matcha powder after a couple of minutes.

Tip the onions into a bowl, add the other burger ingredients and combine thoroughly with your hands. Divide into 4 patties, cover with clingfilm (plastic wrap) and place in the freezer for 10 minutes.

To cook the burgers, heat a little olive oil in a griddle pan until very hot. Add 2 burgers at a time, cooking for 3–4 minutes on each side, depending on how you like your burger. When you flip the burgers, add a slice of cheese, if using, to the top of each so that it melts.

Heat a frying pan (skillet) and add the butter. Once melted, sauté the spinach over a high heat for a minute.

Rest the burgers for a couple of minutes before serving in the brioche buns with onion jam, spinach, avocado and pea shoots or salad leaves.

SWEETS & DRINKS

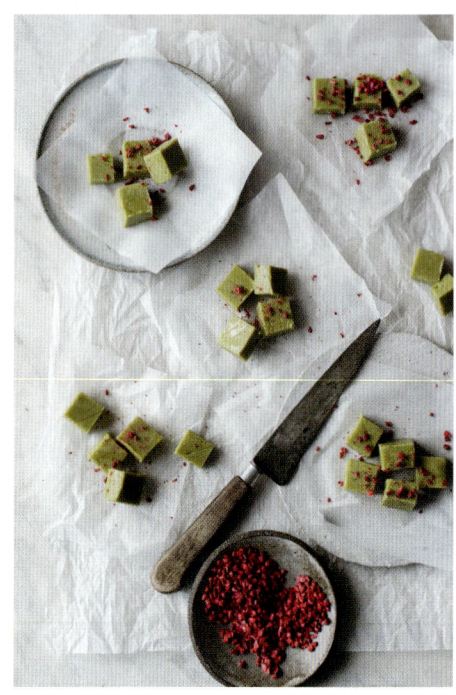

61	**White Chocolate Squares**
63	**Matcha Eton Mess**
64	**Matcha Lemon Posset**
65	**Matcha Chocolate**
66	**Matcha Lollipops**
69	**Shortbread**
70	**Matcha Bliss Balls**
71	**Matcha Tea Loaf**
72	**Matcha Affogato**
75	**Classic Matcha Tea**
76	**Matcha Latte**

MAKES 12 PIECES

WHITE CHOCOLATE SQUARES

This is a buttery, chocolatey treat. As we've said before, matcha goes well with butter, cream and chocolate, so this recipe is definitely worth making to devour on special occasions.

---

60 ml (2½ fl oz) double (heavy) cream
180 g (6½ oz) white chocolate, chopped
15 g (½ oz) salted butter
1 tablespoon matcha powder
pinch of sea salt
dried raspberry pieces, to garnish

Line a 15 cm (6 in) square baking tin with clingfilm (plastic wrap).

Pour the cream into a saucepan and bring almost to boiling point. Remove from the heat and add the chopped chocolate, butter, matcha and salt. Stir well with a rubber spatula until completely combined.

Pour into the lined tin and use the spatula to smooth the surface. Chill in the refrigerator for 3–4 hours, or until firm. Remove from the tin by lifting up the clingfilm, or flip out on to a board. Cut into squares and sprinkle with dried raspberry pieces.

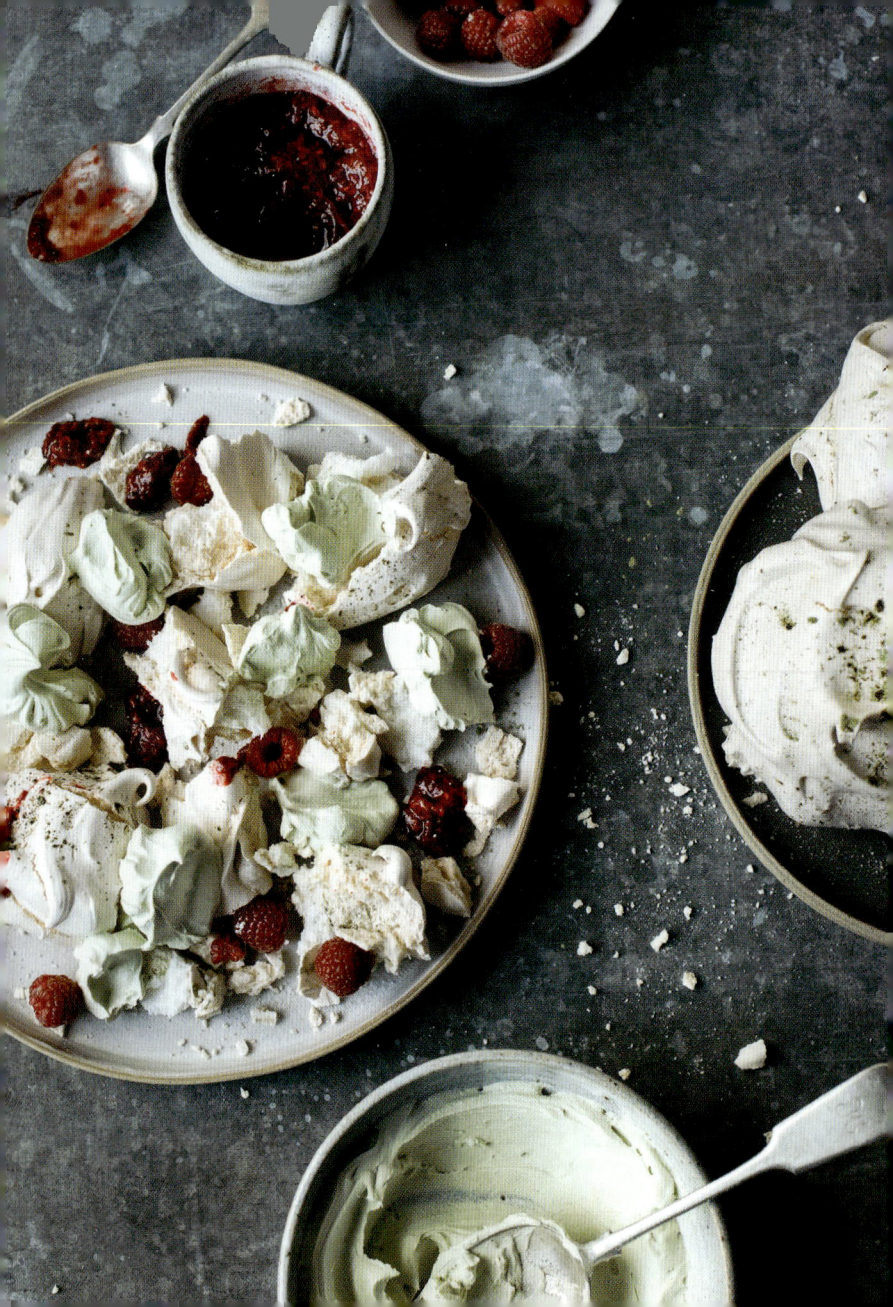

SERVES 4

MATCHA ETON MESS

For an easier version of this, you can use pre-made meringues, but it's even more delicious when you make your own. Prepare the Eton mess on the same day while the meringues are super-fresh.

---

270 g (9¾ oz) raspberries, washed and patted dry
1 teaspoon honey
250 ml (9 fl oz) double (heavy) cream
2 teaspoons matcha powder, plus extra for dusting
20 g (¾ oz) caster (superfine) sugar

FOR THE MERINGUES
1 egg white
pinch of sea salt
230 g (8 oz) caster sugar

Start by making the meringues. Preheat the oven to 140°C (275°F), Gas Mark 1 and line a baking tray with baking paper (parchment).

Put the egg white into a clean bowl with the salt and whisk until they hold soft peaks. Add half the sugar and whisk to blend well. Add the remaining sugar and whisk again until the mixture is thick and shiny and holds stiff peaks.

Dollop large spoonfuls of meringue on to the lined tray, flattening them slightly with the back of the spoon. Bake in the oven for 2 hours, until the meringues are completely dry and crisp on the outside (they will still be a bit squishy in the middle) and can be lifted off the paper easily. Transfer to a wire rack and leave to cool in a dry place.

Blitz 150 g (5½ oz) of the raspberries with the honey in a blender until you have a smooth sauce, then set aside.

Gently whisk the cream, matcha powder and sugar together until it is very lightly whipped.

Break the meringues into bite-sized pieces and place on a serving platter. Top with matcha cream, raspberry sauce and the remaining whole raspberries. Dust with matcha powder before serving.

SERVES 6

MATCHA LEMON POSSET

This is a simple but luxurious dessert, perfect for when you have friends round for dinner.

---

600 ml (20 fl oz) double (heavy) cream
150 g (5½ oz) caster (superfine) sugar
1 vanilla pod, split lengthways
juice of 2 lemons
2 teaspoons matcha powder, or to taste

Pour the cream into a large saucepan and add the sugar and vanilla pod. Bring to the boil, then simmer for 3 minutes. Remove the pan from the heat and whisk in the lemon juice.

Put the matcha powder into a small bowl and whisk in enough of the cream mixture to make a loose paste. Pour this into the pan with the rest of the cream and whisk to combine.

Pour the lemon matcha cream through a sieve (strainer) into a jug, and then pour into 6 ramekin dishes. Leave the mixture to cool, then refrigerate for 6 hours before serving.

MAKES ABOUT 10 SHARDS

MATCHA CHOCOLATE

Matcha goes fantastically with dark chocolate, while the white chocolate in this recipe creates dramatic visual effect.

---

200 g (7 oz) dark chocolate
100 g (3½ oz) white chocolate
1 teaspoon matcha powder
few good pinches of sea salt

Place 2 heatproof bowls over 2 saucepans of gently simmering water, making sure the bases of the bowls don't touch the water in the bottom. Break the dark chocolate into one bowl, the white chocolate and matcha powder into the other. Use spatulas to stir the chocolate until completely melted and smooth.

Line a baking tray with baking paper (parchment) and pour the melted dark chocolate over it, spreading it as evenly as possible using the spatula. Dot the dark chocolate evenly with the matcha white chocolate, then use a cocktail stick to create swirls. Sprinkle over a little sea salt and transfer to the refrigerator to cool for at least 2 hours.

Break the chocolate sheet into shards before serving.

MAKES 6 LOLLIPOPS

MATCHA LOLLIPOPS

The white chocolate is an extra treat here, but use milk or dark chocolate if you prefer. Using ready-made Greek yogurt with honey means that you don't need to add any sweetener, but you can use natural Greek yogurt and add 1–2 tablespoons of honey, according to your taste.

---

500 g (1 lb) Greek yogurt with honey
2 teaspoons matcha powder
½ teaspoon vanilla extract
100 g (3½ oz) white chocolate, broken into pieces
2 teaspoons cacao nibs
2 teaspoons hazelnuts, crushed

Whisk together the Greek yogurt, matcha powder and vanilla extract until thoroughly combined.

Divide the mixture between 6 lolly moulds. Insert a wooden lolly stick into the centre of each mould and freeze for at least 6 hours.

Before serving, melt the chocolate in a heatproof bowl set over a saucepan of barely simmering water. Stir until melted, then set aside.

Take the lolly moulds out of the freezer and hold under the cold tap for a few seconds until you can release the lollies from them. Dip into the melted chocolate or, using a spoon, drizzle the chocolate over the sides. Sprinkle with the cacao nibs and hazelnuts.

Serve as soon as the chocolate sets.

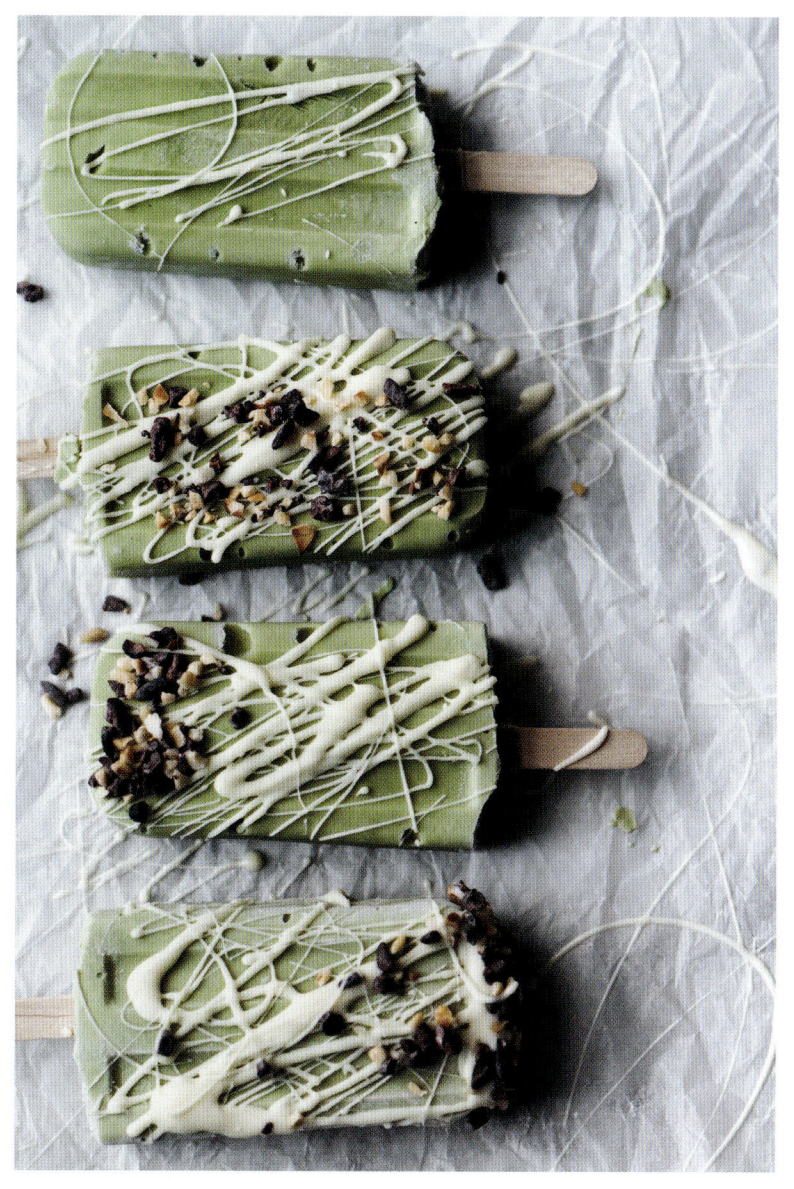

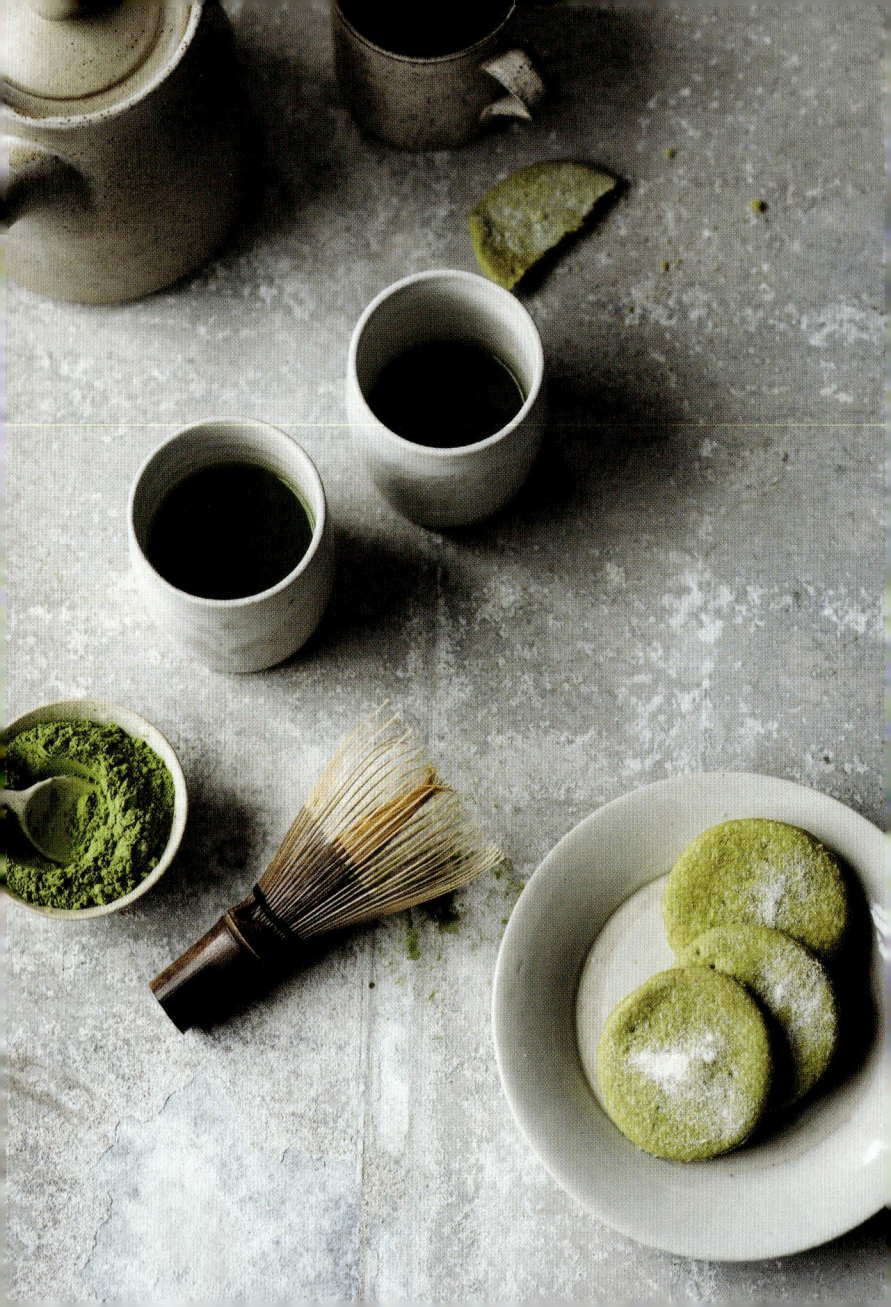

MAKES ABOUT 10 BISCUITS

SHORTBREAD

Matcha and butter are a match made in heaven. The matcha adds a wonderful extra hint of flavour to these crumbly, buttery shortbread biscuits.

---

100 g (3½ oz) unsalted butter, softened, plus extra for greasing
50 g (2 oz) caster (superfine) sugar, plus extra for dusting
100 g (3½ oz) plain (all-purpose) flour
50 g (2 oz) cornflour (cornstarch)
2 teaspoons matcha powder
pinch of sea salt

Lightly butter a baking tray.

Put the butter and sugar in a bowl and use a wooden spoon or hand-held electric mixer to cream until light and fluffy.

Sift the flour and cornflour into a separate bowl and mix in the matcha powder and salt until completely combined. Add this to the creamed butter and mix until smooth.

Tip this mixture on to a lightly floured surface and knead to a dough. Roll out the dough to a thickness of about 1 cm (½ in) and use a round biscuit cutter to cut out circles, placing them on the greased tray. Chill the biscuits on the tray for 30 minutes while you preheat the oven to 180°C (350°F), Gas Mark 4.

Bake the shortbread for 20 minutes, then remove from the oven and leave for a few minutes before transferring to a wire rack and dusting with more caster sugar.

Stored in an airtight container, these biscuits will keep for 3 days.

MAKES 10 BALLS

MATCHA BLISS BALLS

It's actually incredibly easy to make raw energy balls, as all you have to do is blitz everything together. This recipe is also great if you add a couple of teaspoons of raw cacao powder.

---

75 g (3 oz) raw cashew nuts
30 g (1 oz) desiccated (shredded) coconut, unsweetened
120 g (4 oz) dried apple pieces
2 teaspoons matcha powder
½ teaspoon ground ginger
2 tablespoons coconut oil
25 g (1 oz) raw pistachio nuts, shelled and chopped, for rolling

Place all the ingredients, except the pistachios, in a food processor and blend to a paste.

Roll into balls about the size of a walnut, then roll gently in the chopped pistachios.

Chill in the refrigerator for at least 15 minutes before you enjoy.

MAKES 1 LOAF CAKE

MATCHA TEA LOAF

This is a matcha take on a traditional tea loaf, which would usually be made with black tea. The tea is perfect for soaking the fruit so that it is soft, making a lovely moist loaf.

---

350 ml (12 fl oz) water
2 teaspoons matcha powder
350 g (12 fl oz) mixed sultanas and raisins
butter, for greasing
2 eggs, beaten
250 g (8 oz) self-raising flour
200 g (7 oz) soft dark brown sugar
1 teaspoon ground ginger

Boil the water, then leave to cool for 5 minutes. Mix a little of the hot water with the matcha powder to form a loose paste. Add the rest of the water and whisk until combined.

Put the dried fruit into a bowl and pour over the matcha tea. Cover and leave to soak overnight.

Preheat the oven to 180°C (350°F), Gas Mark 4. Grease a loaf tin with a little butter and line with baking paper (parchment).

Add the eggs, flour, sugar and ginger to the fruit mixture and combine well. Pour the mixture into the lined loaf tin, smoothing the surface with a spatula. Bake for 1–1½ hours, until a skewer comes out clean when inserted into the middle of the cake.

Turn the loaf out of the tin and cool on a wire rack. Serve sliced, with butter if you like.

SERVES 4–6

MATCHA AFFOGATO

Affogato is a simple dessert in which ice cream has a liquid – traditionally espresso coffee – poured over it. This matcha version looks even more dramatic and tastes amazing. You can make it even easier and use your favourite ready-made ice cream; it will work just as well with vanilla or coconut.

---

500 ml (17 fl oz) double (heavy) cream
60 g (2¼ oz) chopped stem (preserved) ginger
seeds from 1 vanilla pod
3 tablespoons stem ginger syrup
200 ml (7 oz) classic matcha tea (see page 75)

Pour the cream into a large bowl and use a hand-held electric mixer to whisk it until it forms stiff peaks. Add the ginger, vanilla seeds and syrup, mix well and scrape into a plastic container.

Pop into the freezer for 20 minutes, then take out and stir. Return to the freezer for another hour.

Meanwhile, make your matcha tea and pour into a lovely jug. To serve, scoop the frozen cream into glasses and pour the tea over the top.

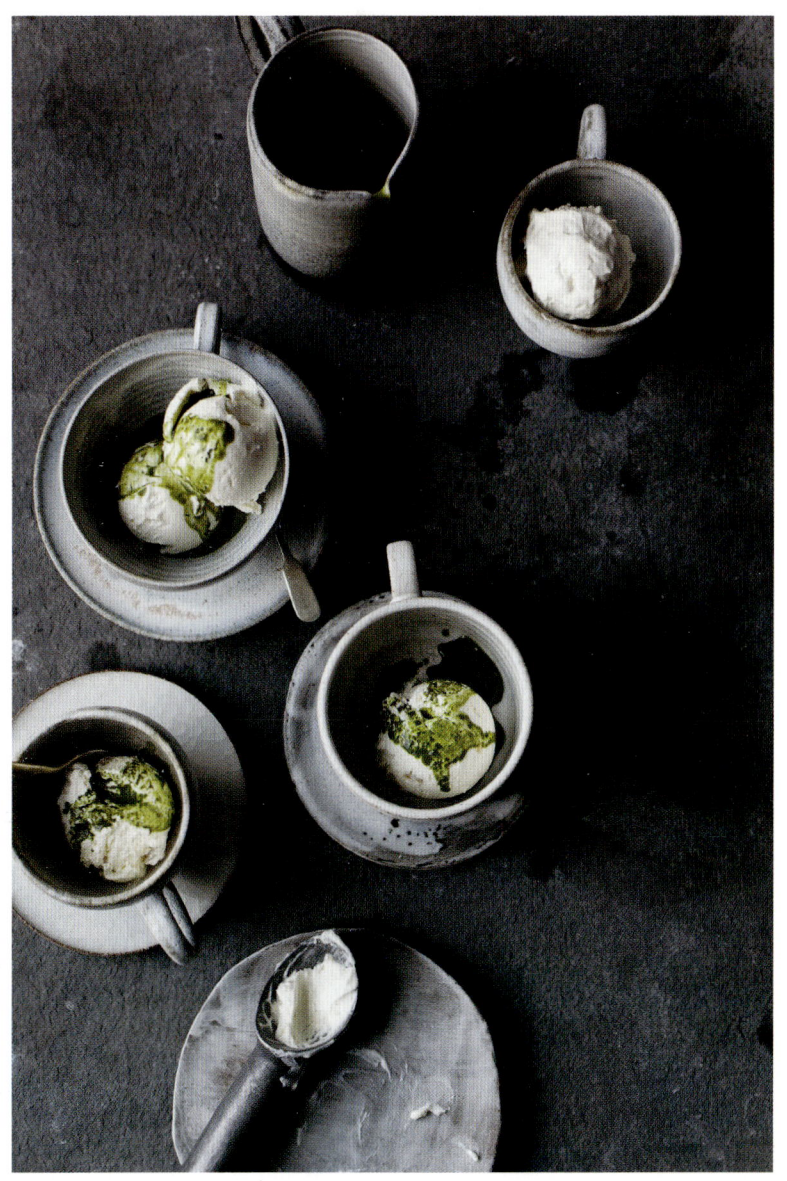

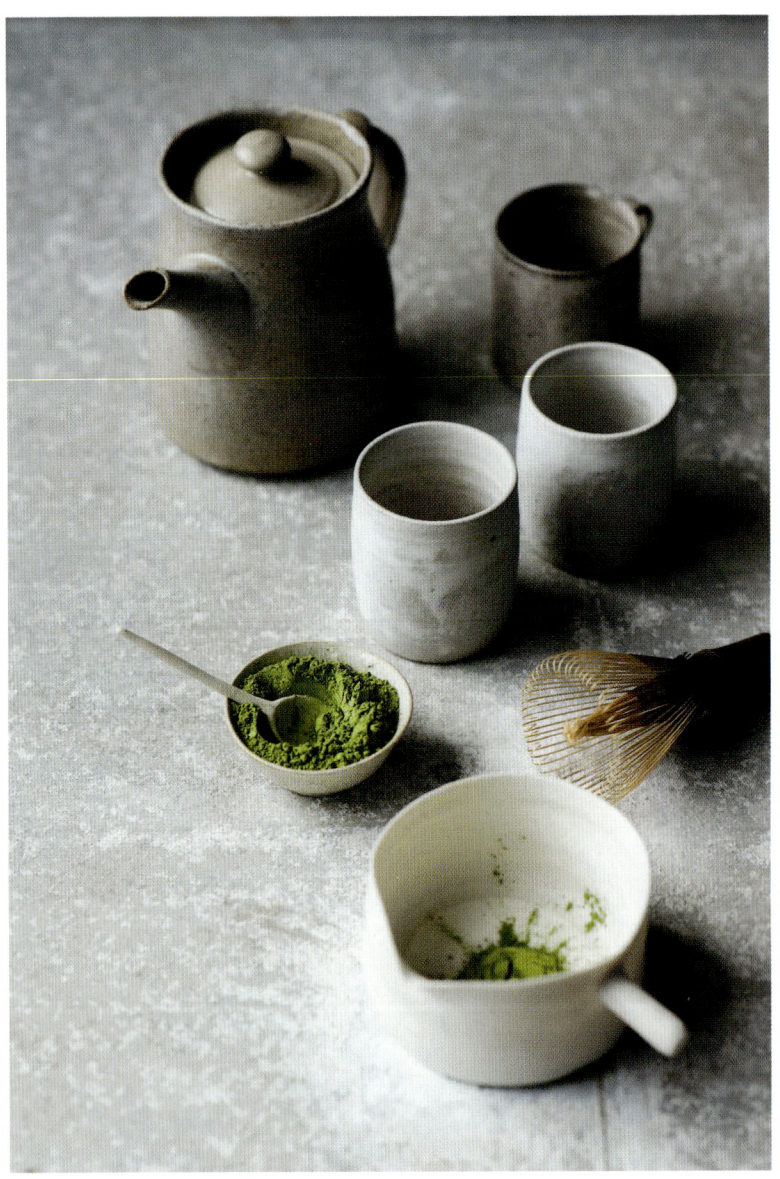

SERVES 1

CLASSIC MATCHA TEA

While the traditional Japanese tea ceremony is very specific and would usually be performed by a special host, there are elements of the ceremony that are worth bringing into your own matcha tea-making. It is a ceremony of mindfulness: in the moment of tea-making all attention is on the tea, it is everything. This is a wonderful practice for being more attentive and engaged in the present, and links perfectly with the idea that matcha aids a mental state of calm alertness. While this helped the Zen monks to meditate, it can also help us to feel both relaxed and focused in our own busy lives. There is also a space for gratitude and appreciation within the ceremony; it reminds us to be thankful for and show respect to even the smallest things, such as a cup of tea.

The exact amount of matcha powder needed will vary, but try to use the ceremonial grade for making the classic tea, which is made by simply whisking it with just-boiled water. Ideally your water should be 80°C (175°F) rather than boiling hot, so allow it to cool a little before making your matcha tea.

1–3 small scoops of matcha powder
200–250 ml (7–8 fl oz) just-boiled water

Add the matcha powder to a bowl or cup, using the traditional scoop – this equates to about ¼–¾ teaspoon. You may need to experiment to find what suits your own taste.

Add a little hot water and whisk in an 'M' shape with a bamboo whisk or small metal whisk.

Once a paste is formed, add the remaining hot water and stir.

Enjoy each sip.

SWEETS & DRINKS

SERVES 1

MATCHA LATTE

Our favourite way to make matcha latte is with almond or oat milk, as both of these alternatives have a natural sweetness to complement the distinct and slightly bitter matcha flavour.

---

200 ml (7fl oz) unsweetened almond or oat milk
½ teaspoon matcha powder, or to taste
1 teaspoon honey (optional)

Heat the almond or oat milk in a small saucepan to a gentle simmer.

In your bowl or cup, add the matcha powder and a little of the hot milk. Whisk until you have a smooth paste. You can then either add the remaining hot milk and froth in the cup using a small hand-held frother, or simmer until frothy in the saucepan, then pour gently into your cup.

Serve with honey if you need a little sweetness.

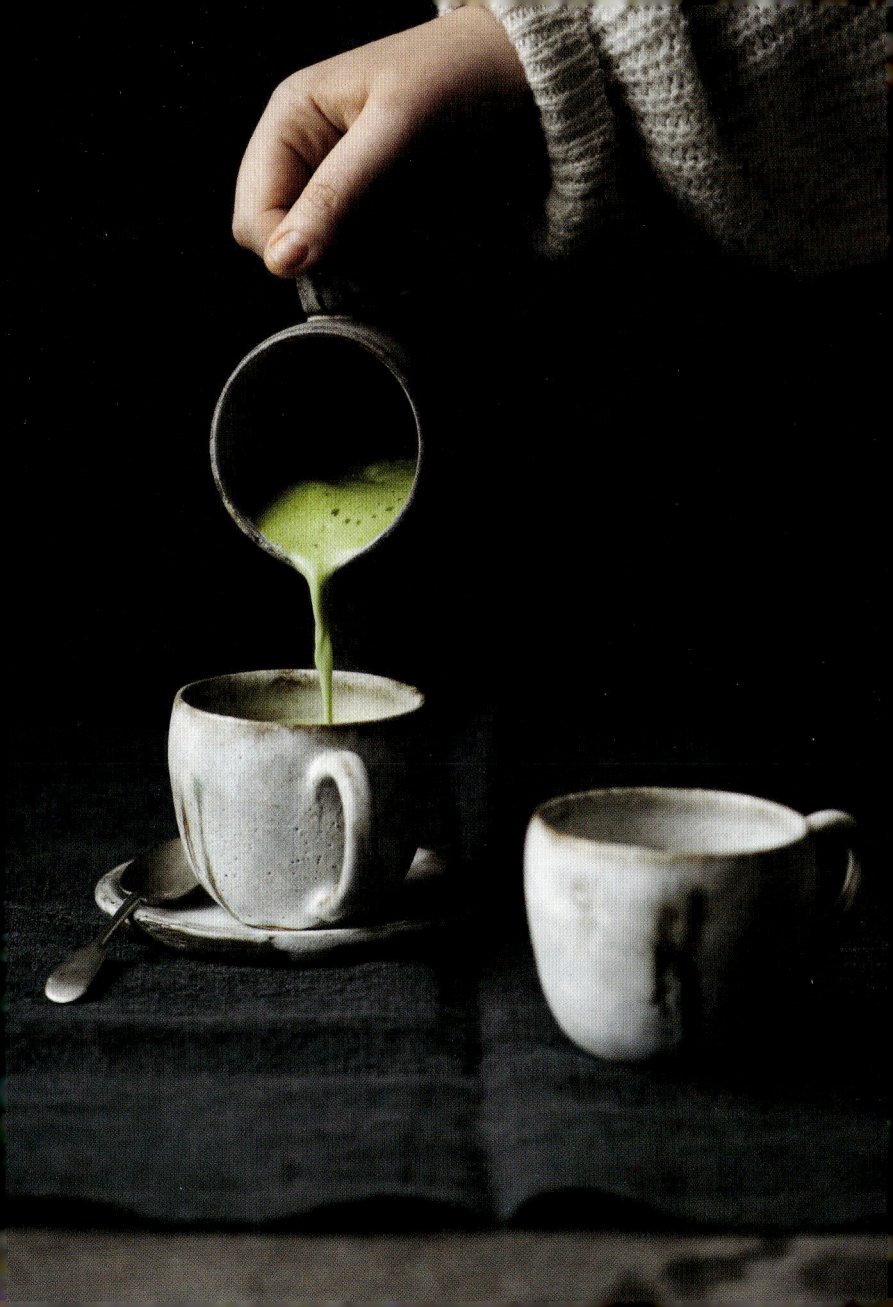

INDEX

affogazto 72
almond butter
   salmon with matcha crumb 53
almond milk
   cauliflower soup with matcha mimosa 29
   matcha latte 76
matcha maple oats 17
apples
   matcha bliss balls 70
apricots
   soda bread 14
asparagus
   matcha poached chicken 56
   asparagus with vinaigrette & quail eggs 38
aubergines
   matcha miso aubergine 39
avocado
   bacon, lettuce & matcha salad 45
   matcha burger 59
   smoothie bowl 13

bacon
   bacon, lettuce & matcha salad 45
   pancakes 18
bananas
   pancakes 18
   smoothie bowl 13
bean sprouts
   ramen 31
beef matcha burger 59
bread
   eggy bread with matcha prawns 22
   matcha burger 59
   soda bread 14
buckwheat
   matcha buckwheat broth 27
butter
   lemon matcha butter 34
   shortbread 69
   sole with matcha beurre blanc & greens 52

cashew nuts
   baked matcha cauliflower 41
   matcha bliss balls 70
cauliflower
   baked matcha cauliflower 41
   cauliflower soup with matcha mimosa 29
cavolo nero
   matcha buckwheat broth 27
   sole with matcha beurre blanc & greens 52
celery
   cauliflower soup with matcha mimosa 29
cheese
   baked matcha cauliflower 41
   cheese & matcha scones 43
   matcha burger 59
   omelette with goats' cheese & herbs 21
   soured cucumber salad with goats' curd 36
chicken
   matcha poached chicken 56
chocolate
   matcha chocolate 65
   matcha lollipops 66
   white chocolate squares 61
coconut
   matcha bliss balls 70
   matcha granola 16
cream
   matcha affogato 72
   matcha Eton mess 63
   matcha lemon posset 64
   scrambled eggs with creamed corn 23
   white chocolate squares 61
cucumber
   smoothie bowl 13
   soured cucumber salad with goats' curd 36

eggs
   bacon, lettuce & matcha salad 45
   cauliflower soup with matcha mimosa 29
   eggy bread with matcha prawns 22

omelette with goats' cheese & herbs	21
scrambled eggs with creamed corn	23
matcha tea loaf	71
pickled eggs	35
ramen	31
asparagus with vinaigrette & quail eggs	38
Eton mess	63

garlic
baked matcha cauliflower	41
pea, mint & matcha soup	32

ginger
matcha affogato	72
matcha buckwheat broth	27

granola — 16

hazelnuts
matcha granola	16
matcha lollipops	66

herbs
omelette with goats' cheese & herbs	21
pea, mint & matcha soup	32
trout with matcha pistachio crumb	50

hummus
matcha & red lentil hummus	33

kale
matcha buckwheat broth	27
sole with matcha beurre blanc & greens	52

latte — 76

leeks
matcha poached chicken	56
pea, mint & matcha soup	32
spiced watercress & matcha soup	25

lemon grass
matcha buckwheat broth	27
matcha noodles with tofu	48
matcha poached chicken	56
summer rolls with matcha dipping sauce	55

lemons
eggy bread with matcha prawns	22
lemon matcha butter	34
matcha lemon posset	64

lentils
matcha & red lentil hummus	33

lettuce
bacon, lettuce & matcha salad	45
summer rolls with matcha dipping sauce	55

limes
omelette with goats' cheese & herbs	21
salad dressing	45
salmon with matcha crumb	53
smoothie bowl	13
trout with matcha pistachio crumb	50

lollipops — 66

mangetout
ramen	31

maple syrup
matcha granola	16
matcha maple oats	17

meringue
matcha Eton mess	63

mint
pea, mint & matcha soup	32

miso
matcha miso aubergine	39

mushrooms
matcha mushroom noodle soup	26
matcha mushroom spelt risotto	47
matcha noodles with tofu	48

noodles
matcha mushroom noodle soup	26
matcha noodles with tofu	48
ramen	31

oats
matcha granola	16
matcha maple oats	17

onions
baked matcha cauliflower	41
matcha burger	59

pak choi
    matcha noodles with tofu   48
pancakes   18
pea, mint & matcha soup   32
pickles   35
pistachio nuts
    matcha bliss balls   70
    trout with matcha pistachio crumb   50

potatoes
    matcha crisps   45
    matcha poached chicken   56
    pea, mint & matcha soup   32
prawns
    eggy bread with matcha prawns   22
    ramen   31
pumpkin seeds
    matcha granola   16
    salmon with matcha crumb   53

quinoa flour
    pancakes   18

raisins
    matcha tea loaf   71
ramen   31
raspberries
    matcha Eton mess   63
    white chocolate squares   61
rice paper wrappers summer rolls with
    matcha dipping sauce   55

salad dressing   45
salmon
    ramen   31
    salmon with matcha crumb   53
    summer rolls with matcha dipping sauce   55
salt
    matcha salt   34

scones
    cheese & matcha scones   43
sea bass
    summer rolls with matcha dipping sauce   55
shortbread   69
smoothie bowl   13
soda bread   14
    sole with matcha beurre blanc & greens   52
spelt
    matcha mushroom spelt risotto   47
spiced watercress & matcha soup   25
spinach
    matcha burger   59
    matcha mushroom noodle soup   26
    smoothie bowl   13
    spiced watercress & matcha soup   25
spring onions
    matcha miso aubergine   39
    ramen   31
sultanas
    matcha tea loaf   71
summer rolls with matcha dipping sauce   55
sweetcorn
    scrambled eggs with creamed corn   23

tea
    classic matcha tea   75
    matcha affogato   72
    matcha tea loaf   71
tofu
    matcha noodles with tofu   48
trout with matcha pistachio crumb   50

vegetables
    pickled vegetables   35
vinaigrette
    asparagus with vinaigrette & quail eggs   38

watercress
    spiced watercress & matcha soup   25

yogurt
    matcha lollipops   66
    pancakes   18
    salad dressing   45
    soda bread   14